Chronic Childhood Disease

An Introduction to
Psychological Theory and Research

CHRISTINE EISER

Department of Psychology
University of Exeter

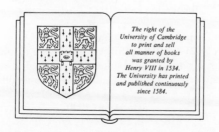

The right of the
University of Cambridge
to print and sell
all manner of books
was granted by
Henry VIII in 1534.
The University has printed
and published continuously
since 1584.

CAMBRIDGE UNIVERSITY PRESS

Cambridge
New York   Port Chester   Melbourne   Sydney

Published by the Press Syndicate of the University of Cambridge
The Pitt Building, Trumpington Street, Cambridge CB2 1RP
40 West 20th Street, New York NY 10011, USA
10 Stamford Road, Oakleigh, Melbourne 3166, Australia

First published 1990

British Library cataloguing in publication data
Eiser, Christine
Chronic childhood disease.
1. Children. Diseases, Psychological aspects.
I. Title
618.9200019

Library of Congress cataloguing in publication data
Eiser, Christine.
Chronic childhood disease: an introduction to psychological
theory and research / Christine Eiser.
p. cm.
Includes bibliographical references.
ISBN 0 521 38519 9. – ISBN 0 521 38682 9 (paperback)
1. Chronic diseases in children – Psychological aspects.
2. Chronic diseases in children – Patients – Family relationships.
I. Title.
RJ380.E37 1990
618.92–dc20   89–71299   CIP

ISBN 0 521 38519 9 hardback
ISBN 0 521 38682 9 paperback

WD

Contents

Preface   page ix

1 *Psychological perspectives in chronic childhood disease*   1
   Introduction   1
   Integration with developmental psychology   3
   Integration of research and clinical practice   6
   Overview   8

2 *Admission to hospital*   11
   Introduction   11
   Psychological impact of admission   14
   Preparation for hospital   17
      Preparation of well children   18
      Evaluations of well child programmes   20
      Preparation of acutely sick children   21
   The role of parents   25
   Conclusions   26

3 *The nature of pain*   28
   Introduction   28
   The measurement and assessment of pain   29
      Distinctions between measurement and assessment   30
      Measurement of pain   30
      Cognitive or self-report methods   30
      Behavioural methods   31
      Physiological methods   33
      Assessment of pain   33

Developmental changes in understanding and experience
  of pain   34
    Definitions and understanding of pain   34
    Symptom-reporting   36
    Coping strategies   36
  Intervention strategies   38
    Relaxation   38
    Puppet therapy   38
    Hypnosis   39
    Coping with stress–inoculation   40
  Conclusions   41

4 *Adjustment in the child with chronic disease*   42

  Introduction   42
  The incidence of 'maladjustment' in chronically sick
    children   44
    Problems of definition   44
    Methodological issues   45
    Theoretical approaches   46
    Population-based research   48
  Asthma   49
  Birth defects   51
  Cancer   51
  Diabetes   53
  Haemophilia   53
  Juvenile rheumatoid arthritis   54
  Renal disease   56
  Sickle-cell anaemia   56
  Spina bifida   57
  Studies involving more than one disease group   57
  Conclusions   58

5 *Adjustment in the family*   61

  Introduction   61
    Knowledge   62
    Variables which determine maternal adjustment   63
  Risk factors   64
    Disease and disability parameters   64
  Resistance factors   67
    Family environment   67
    Social support   68

Marital adjustment   69
General correlates of coping in families   70
Siblings   72
Family communication and interaction   74
Conclusions   76

6   *Communication and education*   78

Introduction   78
The communication of 'bad news'   79
Children's understanding of chronic disease   81
Developmental changes in children's understanding of
    illness   83
The cognitive stage approach to studying children's
    concepts of illness   84
    Concepts of illness   84
    Concepts of the body   85
    Concepts of death   86
    Concepts of related health and illness issues   86
Criticisms of the 'stage' model   88
Alternative theoretical approaches   89
    The 'script' approach   90
Conclusions   91

7   *Intervention programmes*   93

Introduction   93
Programmes to increase disease-related knowledge   93
Programmes to increase self-care skills   95
Programmes to improve social skills   98
Interventions with families and schools   100
    Programmes to improve participation in school-life   100
    Interventions for parents   102
    Interventions with bereaved families   103
Conclusions   104

8   *Coping with chronic disease*   105

Introduction   105
Theoretical approaches to understanding coping during
    childhood   105
Coping with everyday stress   111
    Interpersonal stress   112

    School-related stress   113
  Conclusions   114

9 *Future directions*   116

  Developmental perspectives   116
  Structuralist versus functionalist approaches   118
  The psychological effects of chronic disease on the child   119
    Chronic disease: a single diagnosis?   119
    Outcome measures   121
    Intelligence   121
    Social development   122
    Personality   123
  Other issues in child adjustment research   123
    Time   123
    Gender   124
    Adjustment in families   125
  Psychology–paediatric liaison   126

  References   128

  Author index   159
  Subject index   170

Preface

Recent years have seen a substantial increase in research concerned with the psychological effects of chronic disease on children and their families. This has been reflected in the popularity of journals specifically concerned with child health (e.g. Journal of Pediatric Psychology; Journal of Developmental and Behavioral Pediatrics), the organisation of a number of major conferences (e.g. the Florida conferences on Child Health Psychology in 1988 and 1989) and the publication of a number of important books. Many of these, however, seem to be directed toward those who are active researchers, and are not necessarily appropriate for students newly introduced to the concepts and issues of child health psychology. This book is directed primarily at these groups, and will hopefully appeal equally to students of psychology, medicine, nursing and other disciplines involved in the care of chronically sick children.

I increasingly feel that there should be greater collaboration between researchers and clinicians, and that this is important both to improve the quality of research and to effect change in clinical practice. In addition, I would like to see 'child health psychology' truly developmental, rather than embedded in adult perspectives. Both these themes are central in this book.

I am especially lucky at Exeter in being able to work happily with all the paediatric and nursing staff, and am grateful to them all. Special thanks are due to Dr John Tripp, who is always highly supportive and encouraging. I am also grateful to Dick Eiser, both in his capacity as husband and Head of Department, for his help and constructive advice. At various times, I have been supported financially by the Department of Health and Social Security, the Medical Research Council, the Nuffield Foundation and the Economic and Social Science Research Council. Without this support, this book would not have been written. Finally, I would like to thank Sandy Salisbury for her careful typing of the manuscript.

Christine Eiser
February 1990

I

Psychological perspectives in chronic childhood disease

Introduction

The diagnosis of chronic disease in children sets the stage for a revolution in the way of life experienced by patient and family. Implications are far-reaching, affecting everyday routines, hopes and ambitions and the relationships both between family members and with the outside world. Few families on diagnosis realise the extent to which chronic disease will change every aspect of their lives. This book is concerned with some of these changes, and what is understood about how children and families learn to integrate the restrictions of disease and treatment with other, more routine, aspects of their lives. Chronic disease creates a variety of difficulties with both practical and emotional implications. Some of the more routine aspects of child-care become more complicated, time-consuming and emotionally-laden. For example, all children go through 'difficult' phases, when they may refuse to eat, play with food or are generally messy and disruptive at meal-times. Parents naturally find this very trying, but are often able to deal with the situation by ignoring the mess. Most children eat readily enough when they are hungry, and when they realise that parents are not making an issue of the problem. However, parental anxiety about the chronically sick child can lead to much greater insistence that food be eaten, and a situation therefore develops involving greater conflict. A commonly experienced and irritating aspect of child-rearing becomes a more major family crisis.

Treatments also can disrupt family life. It may be necessary for the child to have medications at specified times, and this may result in interruptions in play or family activities. Simple procedures like taking pills can assume monumental importance if the child is uncooperative or frankly finds it difficult to swallow. Other treat-

Table 1.1. *Incidence and survival data for eleven childhood chronic diseases; adapted from Gortmaker (1985)*

Disease	Age of onset	Typical incidence per 1000 live births	Survival estimates
Cystic fibrosis	variable; most in first year	0.50	70% to 21 years
Spina bifida	birth	1.00	45% to 4–8 years
Leukaemia	maximum onset	0.03	40–60% survival
Congenital heart disease	88% by first year	8.00	52% to 15 years
Asthma	variable; first 1–2 years is normal	10.00	similar to normal
Sickle-cell anaemia	latter part of first year	0.36	95% to 20 years
Chronic kidney disease	variable; 1–15 years	2.00	with treatment, few children die
Juvenile diabetes	peak at 12 years	0.40	95% to 20 years
Muscular dystrophy	after 3 years	0.14	25% to 20 years
Haemophilia	90% by 3–4 years	0.13	relatively normal to 20 years
Cleft palate	birth	0.40	normal

ments, like physiotherapy, can be very time-consuming, even when everyone is being highly cooperative and helpful.

Parents' perceptions and attitudes toward the child can also be affected. The marital relationship may be strained by increased care-taking, and sometimes by anxiety and guilt about the cause of the child's disease. Social life can be restricted, especially if parents feel that no competent child-care is available. Family activities, also, can be more difficult to organise, and consequently everybody comes to lead a restricted life.

Although most chronic diseases are relatively rare, together they affect a significant proportion of children. The total incidence of chronic disease is in the order of 10.0%, although the severity with which children are affected varies enormously. The most common is asthma, which accounts for approximately half of childhood chronic diseases. The incidence of other diseases is shown in Table 1.1. Some of those with asthma, for example, may suffer from occasional bouts of wheeziness which are little more than irritating. At the other end of the spectrum, children may suffer from severe daily (or more frequent) attacks, which require aggressive medication and hospitalisation. While other diseases do not generally show such a range of severity, they vary in terms of specific restrictions that are imposed on the child. For example, some diseases (such as juvenile arthritis or muscular dystrophy) are associated with restricted physical mobility, while others impose no systematic physical restrictions. The child may sometimes feel tired and withdraw from physical activity for this reason, but this is not an on-going problem. Other diseases may be life-threatening (such as leukaemia or other cancers) and become restricting in terms of emotional distress. In addition, these children may be differentially vulnerable to common childhood complaints, and restrictions can follow from attempts to protect them from potentially contagious situations. In some diseases, the child's condition may be relatively stable; others follow a more cyclical course. Again, in leukaemia, periods of health and relative stability can be followed by periods of relapse and more aggressive treatments.

Chronic diseases are conditions that affect children for extended periods of time, often for life. These diseases can be 'managed' to the extent that a degree of pain control or reduction in attacks (of asthma), bleeding episodes (in haemophilia) or seizures (in epilepsy) can generally be achieved. However, they cannot be cured. (An exception is leukaemia and some other cancers, in which it increasingly seems possible that some children may be completely cured.) This book is concerned with how children and their families organise and manage their lives in the face of the demands and restrictions of such chronic diseases. Although many of the difficulties are also experienced by families of physically and mentally handicapped children, and those affected by sensory disorders, the focus of this book is essentially on the effects of chronic disease.

Integration with developmental psychology

There are two themes underlying the review of literature in this book. The first is that research concerned with psychological aspects of chronic disease should be better integrated within general developmental psychology. The second is that there should also be better integration between research work and clinical practice.

There is much lip-service paid to the significance of developmental issues in determining children's adjustment to chronic disease, the effectiveness of communication between medical staff,

parents and children, compliance with treatment or ability to understand medical concepts. While many researchers advocate the need
for a developmental approach, fewer really integrate developmental
concepts into their work. At best, chronological age is used as a gross
indicator of developmental level, but other, perhaps more acceptable
indicators (e.g. reasoning ability) are rarelyused. Some researchers
have used developmental 'stage' as determined by tests of conservation, but this does not satisfactorily take account of objections and
criticisms that have been made regarding stage approaches to
development (see Chapter 6). It is clear that children differ from
adults in their understanding of illness concepts, and in their experience of health, illness and medical care. It is essential that these
differences are an integral part of approaches to the management of
sick children, but they are unlikely to correlate simply with chronological age.

A number of issues are central to research concerned with children
with chronic disease, and to developmental psychology more generally. Despite this overlap in interest, the two lines of research invariably have developed quite independently.

For example, being admitted to hospital is potentially stressful for
children and adults alike, although there is an assumption that
enforced separation from parents is an additional source of distress
for young children. Issues of attachment and separation have traditionally been key issues in developmental psychology.

Similarly, the way in which children respond to chronic disease
appears to be influenced by (a) characteristics of the disease (whether
it is life-threatening, restricts movements, limits social activities or
experiences, etc.); (b) characteristics of the child (age, gender,
personality or coping-style); and (c) characteristics of the family
(problem-solving abilities or communication skills). Again, issues of
child personality and family functioning are central to much
developmental psychology.

The question that has been most thoroughly researched concerns
the effects of chronic disease on children and their families. There has
been an assumption behind most of this work that there is a simple
correlation between severity of disease and adverse psychological
repercussions. The lack of real integration between the two areas has
resulted in an over-simplification in many instances. In studying the
effects of chronic disease on the child, researchers may fall back on
very established measures of IQ, without considering alternative
measures (of memory or reasoning, for example) that might be differentially affected by chronic disease. The massive literature con-

cerned with interviewer effects on obtained IQ scores, or the relationship between IQ and achievement, is generally ignored. As a result, inappropriate measures can be used, and invalid interpretations made.

A second, related example concerns the effects of chronic disease on healthy family members. Again, there is generally assumed to be a simple correlation between the presence of a child with chronic disease and adverse repercussions for others. This is very much reflected in work concerned with healthy siblings, who are often reported to show behavioural and emotional deficits, resent the sick child and react in terms of anger and hostility. Very recently, work by Dunn (1987; 1988; largely concerned with relationships between healthy siblings) has been instrumental in clarifying our understanding of the intricacies of sibling relationships. There is no advantage in seeing the relationship predominantly in terms of hostility and aggression. Rather, the sibling relationship needs to be seen as an important precursor of adult relationships. Through their siblings, children learn to mediate parental influence, and derive a great deal of mutual support and benefit. Research concerned with the effects of chronic disease on healthy siblings needs to take account of this range of behaviours and emotions, rather than be restricted to the rather narrow perspective which had traditionally been adopted.

Children with chronic disease are, first and foremost, children. With healthy children, they share similar concerns and anxieties: about their relationships with other children, with siblings and parents, about their abilities to succeed and about hopes, dreams and ambitions. They fluctuate in their desires to be part of the family, to be a child and nurtured, while at the same time wishing to be independent and free from parental restrictions. The focus on chronic disease as the key influence is essentially inadequate, because it fails to acknowledge the role of variables other than chronic disease, on adjustment and relationships.

First, it means that no account has been taken of the implications of disease for normal developmental growth. It is acknowledged that the adolescent with chronic disease faces special problems in establishing independence from parents because of the restrictions of disease and help that may be required with treatments. Many adolescents experience considerable turmoil and may reject treatments during this period. A focus on the disease has resulted in the view that this is essentially pathological behaviour. An alternative perspective, and one which has roots in normal developmental theory, is more likely to relate these difficulties of adolescence to

normal behaviour: a reflection of a healthy (albeit somewhat incon-
venient and troublesome) aspect of growing up. Very different
implications for intervention follow from these two perspectives:
the one seeing the adolescent's behaviour as pathological or disturbed, and the other attributing it to normal processes.

The second problem with focusing exclusively on the psychological effects of disease is that the work is theoretically and methodologically limited. Research concerned with children's understanding of disease, for example, is entrenched in a stage view of development. Children's beliefs about illness are seen to develop in a series
of systematic stages, paralleling development of concepts such as
space, time or conservation. Little account has ever been taken of the
criticisms that have been made of stage models, and certainly no
efforts have been directed at explaining how children proceed from
one stage to the next. Neither has account been taken of the fact that
there is less empirical evidence concerning stage-bound behaviour
than was previously supposed.

In parallel with this emphasis on the stage model of development
rather than any other are restrictions in terms of available methodologies. A great deal of data has been derived from semi-structured
interviews with children about disease-related attitudes or
behaviours. This emphasis has restricted the data-base to children of
reasonable verbal abilities and generally also to those of school-age.
These verbal methods are inappropriate for younger children, and
for those with more limited verbal and interpersonal skills. Little
ingenuity has been shown by researchers in employing alternative
methods of data-collection. Greater awareness of developmental
psychology and associated innovations in research methods are
crucial to improving methodologies and the scope of our understanding about children's reasoning about illness.

In summary then, accounts of the psychological effects of chronic
disease on children and their families need to be integrated within a
developmental framework. The emphasis needs to shift away from
the identification of psycho-pathology and malfunction. The problems faced by children and their families need to be understood in
terms of models that recognise the potential difficulties and coping
resources available to people managing very special circumstances.

Integration of research and clinical practice

The second theme in this book relates to the distinction that is often
drawn between research concerned with chronic disease in children

and clinical practice. The distinction arises for many reasons. First and foremost, researchers and clinicians differ in training. From this basic difference arise divergences in attitudes, theoretical orientations, methodological and statistical skills and perceived priorities. The researcher is trained to collect information from a large number of children (having 'matched' those with chronic disease with healthy individuals of similar age, gender, background, etc.), and then to look for similarities within and between the groups using statistical methods. The researcher can be disdainful about clinical case studies, arguing that these are not necessarily representative of sick children as a whole, and that implications cannot be drawn from single case studies to all children suffering from a chronic disease. In contrast, the clinician can be sceptical about the value of statistical studies, arguing that important individual differences are lost.

There are, of course, merits and limitations in both approaches. The merit of research work is that it is possible to make generalisations about how individuals respond in a given situation. Given a research finding that a sizeable proportion of children with chronic disease under-achieve in school, it is perhaps easy to justify remedial help for all such children, whereas this is more difficult if only one child is known to have educational difficulties. It is helpful for parents to see their child's school difficulty as natural and commonly experienced, rather than as a reflection of the child's limited abilities or an unexpected consequence of the illness or its treatment. Either of these latter implications might be drawn from a narrowly clinical perspective.

A disadvantage of a more statistical approach, however, is that it is possible to lose sight of the child's special circumstances. It is easier for researchers to distance themselves from intense emotional experiences and remain aloof from the problem of providing real and practical help. Clinicians may make a more honest attempt at this. However, the interventions they offer may be of a trial-and-error nature, or focus exclusively on a preferred theoretical background. Clinicians do not always stand back from their work and ask if their methods really are associated with any success, or whether improvements could be achieved by better matching of therapy, patient and problem.

Neither researchers nor clinicians have exclusive rights to work with chronically sick children. However, both groups have an obligation to collaborate and offer a more substantial service to children and families. This book is essentially about research findings and issues, although the implications for clinical practice are extensive. By drawing together this literature, it is hoped that the relevance of this work for clinical practice is clearly defined and easily extrapolated.

Notwithstanding these criticisms, it is possible to point to considerable achievements in research so far. At the very least, it is now generally acknowledged that chronic disease is a potentially threatening event for children and their families, and that the success of paediatric medicine should be measured, not simply in terms of survival, but also in terms of the psychological consequences. The degree to which research findings have had direct implications for care and management of sick children is variable, but not completely insignificant.

Overview

Most children with chronic disease are admitted to hospital, invariably on diagnosis and then at intermittent intervals depending on the condition. Although current practice (at least in North America and Great Britain) is to reduce the incidence and duration of hospital stays as far as possible, the majority of those with chronic disease experience a greater number of admissions than healthy children. The atmosphere on paediatric wards has changed substantially since the publication of the Platt report in 1959 (Platt Committee, Great Britain, 1959). Nevertheless, hospital is still a potentially threatening environment for many children. Aside from practical improvements that have been made (for example, allowing parents unrestricted visiting time and encouraging play and social activities on the ward), the second, more recent innovation has involved attempts to prepare children for admission and treatment. In Chapter 2, different intervention techniques are assessed and compared.

A major criticism to emerge is that interventions have not been developed for groups most in need (the chronically sick, very young or mentally retarded children). Insufficient attention has been paid to developmental changes in children's understanding of hospital and medical treatment, specific concerns about these issues, and learning abilities.

Similar criticisms can be made about interventions developed specifically to help children manage painful procedures. Children with chronic disease often experience more than their fair share of invasive and highly painful treatments. Many assumptions about the nature of childhood pain have dominated clinical practice. These include assumptions that children feel less pain than adults because of incomplete myelination or heightened pain thresholds. As it becomes increasingly acknowledged that there is no evidence for these assumptions, attempts to help children manage pain have mushroomed. Some of these are reviewed in Chapter 3.

It is very easy to point to a whole range of practical and emotional difficulties that chronically sick children may experience. Research concerned with the psychological impact of chronic disease has been dominated by efforts to understand development within this adverse framework. In Chapter 4, the ramifications of chronic disease for educational achievement, and social and emotional behaviour, are considered. Most research is necessarily limited to considering immediate or very short-term effects, although increasingly it is possible to question whether or not chronic disease is associated with deficits into adulthood. Increasingly, too, it seems inadequate to consider all children with chronic disease as a homogeneous group. Children with certain diseases, especially those involving physical, sensory or intellectual deficits, appear to have a poorer prognosis in terms of psychological development. At a practical level, this research points to the potential value of making remedial help available on a routine basis to all chronically sick children.

This work concerned with adjustment in children with chronic disease is paralleled by work concerned with adjustment in their families. However, 'families' is used in a very restricted sense. Mothers are assumed to shoulder the major burden of care-taking and to be generally more emotional than fathers. In Chapter 5, it is suggested that there are few grounds for these assumptions; very little is known about the role of fathers in families of sick children. Again, research has concentrated on identifying the adverse effects of the disease on maternal adjustment, at the expense of understanding changes in parenting, discipline and expectations. A related assumption is that family adjustment is associated with the child's adjustment; in particular poorly adjusted families have poorly adjusted children. There may be a degree of truth in this, but the mechanisms whereby this occurs are far from understood. Nevertheless, there is a clear implication that interventions directed at either child or family, without taking into account the interactions between them, are unlikely to be successful.

In Chapter 6, the question of how illness and treatment is explained to children is considered. Again, there is a non-substantiated assumption that 'good' communication about the diagnosis is important to ensure the child's cooperation and compliance with treatment. In fact, many factors influence compliance (for example, the complexity of the treatment schedule, the attitudes of family and friends), and the role of communication should not be over-emphasised. It is generally argued that attempts to explain illness to children should take account of development factors. These explanations need also to take into account social and cultural factors as well as the role of illness experience, in addition to the child's age.

Certainly, a developmental framework does not form the basis of most intervention work. For the most part, interventions have been developed for adult populations, and these then extrapolated for work with children. While this may be satisfactory at one level, it is only one way to proceed. More interventions need to be developed based on specific childhood problems. Interventions with chronically sick children are often intended to increase knowledge, promote effective self-care techniques and, more recently, to encourage self-confidence and assertiveness in dealing with others and explaining the limitations of the disease. While many interventions are highly original, innovative and have the welfare of the child clearly in mind, evaluations sadly lack methodological rigour. It is almost impossible to make even gross generalisations about the relative efficacies of different procedures.

Finally, in Chapter 8 the emphasis becomes much more positive, considering adaptive coping strategies that may be associated with coping with both disease-related and more everyday common stresses. Developmental changes in the appraisal of stressful situations, and the resources and strategies available, are considered. It is emphasised that children cope, not only with stresses associated with their disease, but also with a host of others which are experienced by all children. These stresses stem from situations at school, at home, and with friends or strangers. The strategies that children rely on to deal with their disease are based on those that they have learned to use successfully in other contexts. The psychological repercussions of chronic disease are intimately bound up with developments in this wider context.

2

Admission to hospital

Introduction

How do you think you would feel if you were told you had to go into hospital next week? Chances are you would feel a bit apprehensive: concerned about what might be wrong and what the treatment would be. But you might well feel as much concern about the fact that you would be forced to miss some course-work and would fall behind others. You might also resent the fact that you would be in hospital on the same day as you had planned to see an important match, or would be unable to go to a party that promised to be particularly good. You would resent the disruption in everyday work and social life.

These sorts of things concern children too, especially those of school-age. Children due to take important public exams may well feel highly anxious about the repercussions of missing school. Younger children have their concerns too. They are unlikely to know their way around hospitals; the whole environment is very alien. The endless lengths of corridors and sheer size of modern hospitals can be daunting to a child (and parent) – however do people find their way around? There are masses of personnel to cope with as well: admissions officers, porters, domestics, nurses (of all grades), medical students, housemen, consultants, radiographers, physiotherapists, social workers, psychologists even – just exactly what do they all do? Over and above all this, children have very idiosyncratic and practical concerns. For many, it will be the first time they have spent a night away from home, away from a familiar environment and trusted adults. All children worry about how they will fit into hospital routines. Will someone read a bedtime story? Will they be allowed to take teddy? Will there be a light over their bed, or will they have to sleep in the dark? Will they be given milk and biscuits as at home? Where abouts is the toilet? For young children, these are very real concerns that need to be addressed. And we haven't yet touched on anxieties associated with the treatment itself: what will the doctor do? Will it hurt? What *is* an operation?

Children can have quite distorted views about what goes on in hospitals, what doctors do and what medical treatment involves (Steward & Steward, 1981; Redpath & Rogers, 1984; Eiser & Patterson, 1983). For example, healthy children of 5 years or less may think that hospital is where you go to become ill, rather than get better. They may think that people stay in hospital for years and years, and that they rarely (if ever) come out alive. Their experience and knowledge is likely to be based on the fact that a grand-parent was once taken to hospital, and then never seen again. This may result in a child feeling that hospitals are rather sinister places.

As they grow up, children become more knowledgeable about what happens in hospital. Their knowledge may not always be entirely accurate, however, based on information gleaned from soap operas on television, or rather dramatic accounts given by peers. The latter can be quite alarmist; having survived hospital admission and treatment, a child likes to recount the experience with much bravado!

An alternative, and just as popular image of hospital among 7–8 year olds is that they are rather boring places.

'Oh', Apis told me, 'they leave people here for weeks before they touch them. We've seen children very nearly die of boredom in here. In this very ward.' (Keneally, 1978)

There is not much to do, and also hospitals are places where things *hurt*. Again, this view is perpetuated in children's books. For example, Roald Dahl (1986) gives a very gruesome account of the removal of his tonsils and adenoids. The operation, performed in 1924, was conducted without anaesthetic. Dahl, 'seduced' by the doctor's quiet voice, opened his mouth, and watched as a mass of flesh and blood was twisted from the back of his throat. Immediately afterwards, he walked the full half-hour journey home.

Parents and medical staff like to assure children that treatment does not hurt, but in fact it often does, and it may be more honest to say so. Older children become increasingly adult-like in their under-standing of what happens in hospital, but even adolescents have needs quiet distinct from those of adults. Adolescents do not want to be treated like babies; they do not altogether fit in well on the adult ward either. On the paediatric ward, the adolescent may resent the noise and disorder, but on the adult ward, the adolescent can be unnecessarily exposed to stress and suffering. The adolescent is neither child nor adult and this is as much a dilemma in the hospital ward as it is in everyday life.

It is unfortunate that doctors and nurses are responsible for much of the pain that is inflicted on children in hospital. It is doctors and nurses who give injections, and all the other traumatic procedures, and they can seem very cold and calculating about it. In all probability, it may be the 50th time the doctor has done a lumbar puncture,[1] and that can make him or her seem rather blasé about it, but for the child it is a major event, and cannot be dismissed lightly. If it is the doctor's *first* lumbar puncture, it may well be that his or her concerns are not predominantly with the child. Rather, the doctor is likely to be concerned about personal anxieties: getting the procedure right and not needing to ask a more senior colleague for help. Personal anxieties about the work may blind a doctor to the impact of the procedure on the child.

For whatever reason, children can come to believe that doctors and nurses deliberately inflict pain, and even enjoy doing it. Brewster (1982) studied 50 children with chronic disease who had experienced a considerable amount of hospitalisation and treatment. She found that many 5-year-olds thought that doctors deliberately set out to hurt them. Children of 7–8 years accepted that doctors did not mean to hurt, but believed that they did not care. Children of about 11 years of age thought that doctors realised that they hurt children, but were unaware of how much they hurt unless they had also experienced the treatment themselves. Brewster also found that the more medical treatment children experienced, the more entrenched these views became. That is, the more experienced they were with doctors, the more definite they were that doctors deliberately and callously inflicted pain and suffering. Sometimes, when young patients seem particularly difficult and uncooperative, it is worth putting yourself in their positions for a short while. Children's mistrust of the medical profession builds up over a period of time; their resentment may be the result of many previous experiences with apparently uncaring professionals.

What doctors actually do to patients in the interests of making them better can be quite difficult for the child to understand. Children may be aware that they have an acute pain in their stomach, yet

---

[1] A needle is inserted into the spinal column. Spinal fluid is withdrawn for analysis and drugs injected as a prophylactic treatment to reduce the risk of central nervous system disease or relapse.

doctors insist on giving an injection in the arm, or making them swallow foul-tasting medicine. How can an injection in the arm make their stomach better? Sometimes, too, children go to the doctor feeling perfectly well, and come away feeling terrible. This applies particularly to children with chronic disease, leukaemia for example. Children in remission may come to out-patients feeling fine, and go away after a bone-marrow aspiration[2] feeling very sick. For children with leukaemia this experience can go on for years; it is no wonder some grow to resent the medical profession and all that is associated with it.

Psychological impact of admission

Most reviews on the effects of hospitalisation on children begin by stating that admission can be a traumatic experience. Certainly the older literature very much supported this view. Research in the 1950s showed that admission was often highly distressing, and could have long-lasting adverse repercussions. In Great Britain, Bowlby (1960), as well as Robertson (1952; 1958), conducted some exemplary work. As a result of their research, the Robertsons made a film called *A two-year-old goes to hospital*. It is still available, and makes impressive viewing. A two-year-old girl is admitted for a routine hernia operation. Her mother is shown leaving the distressed child, clearly assured by the nurse that the child would settle down as soon as she was left. The child first objects violently, but over the 10-day stay, her mood changes dramatically. By the end of her stay in hospital, the child is clearly withdrawn and depressed.

Over the last 20 or 30 years, there has been a great deal of research showing that hospital admission can have serious adverse effects on the child's psychological well-being, at least in the short-term. Further, children subject to frequent or long admissions, and those from less privileged backgrounds, are especially at risk (Douglas, 1975; Quinton & Rutter, 1976). Frequent, and multiple admissions may be associated with longer-term emotional and behavioural difficulties. No single explanation of why hospital is so stressful is possible. Hospital admission creates a number of stresses for the child: the stress of separation from parents, the pain of treatment, the unfamiliarity of the environment and the fear of the unknown (Rachman & Phillips, 1975).

---

[2] A needle is inserted into the child's hip-bone. Bone marrow is withdrawn to be tested for the presence of cancer cells.

Since the 1960s there has been a concerted effort to improve life on a paediatric ward. In Great Britain, these changes can be primarily attributed to two events. The first was the publication of the Platt report in 1959. The government report made a number of practical suggestions to improve care of hospitalised children. Most notably, it recommended that:

(1) All children should be nursed on paediatric wards, and that staff should be specially trained to nurse children.
(2) Provision should be made for the child to have access to educational and recreational activities.
(3) Parents should be entitled to unrestricted visits to their children, and provision should also be made for parents to stay in hospital overnight with their child.

The implementation of these recommendations can be largely credited to a voluntary organisation, the National Association for the Welfare of Children in Hospital (NAWCH), established in 1961. The extent to which all the recommendations are reflected in the practice of a particular hospital is still highly variable. Even within the same hospital, procedures can vary from ward to ward. Nevertheless, it is clear that hospital admission for a child today is considerably better than was offered to previous generations. These improvements are reflected in three recently published surveys: two in the United States (Azarnoff & Woody, 1981; Peterson & Ridley-Johnson, 1980) and one in England (Thornes, 1983).

Some reluctance to initiate changes on paediatric wards can be attributed to both parents and staff. Many medical staff did not feel that parents had a place in a hospital ward, and assumed only that they would be in the way and reduce the efficiency with which the ward could be run. Such people also viewed with horror the idea of children being able to paint, or play with sand and water, and generally make a mess in hospital.

Neither did all parents welcome the idea of being able to stay with their child. These parents were often terrified of hospitals themselves. Others were torn between what they saw as their duties to the sick child, and duties to others at home – husband and other children. Also for parents, staying in hospital can be extremely depressing. They are in an unfamiliar environment without the structure of a routine day at home. There may be little to do. They may be forced into close proximity with other parents, some of whom are not people they would normally choose to interact with. Bitterness can build up between parents, especially where children are seriously ill.

In these cases, parents can be forced together for long periods of time, and a kind of competition can develop between them over their children's health. They will discuss and compare all aspects of the children's treatment, and this can result in misunderstanding and confusion.

Sometimes, parents can be a nuisance on the ward. They can also be an asset. It is an ideal opportunity for parents to learn about their child's treatment, especially important if the child has a chronic condition which requires the parents to assume much responsibility on discharge home. Parents can also do much to reassure the child. They provide a continuity between home and hospital life, and generally help by dealing with the adult world of the hospital on the child's behalf (Consumers Association, 1980). Often, too, parents can be a source of support to each other.

Play-leaders and teachers, too, are essential to the smooth running of the paediatric ward. Again, one of the main tasks is ensuring continuity between home and hospital. Also, both play-leaders and teachers are in an ideal position to find out particular concerns that the child has about treatment, and offer some assurances in a language that the child is most likely to understand.

There have therefore been a number of innovations in the organisation of paediatric wards. The question is, have these really resulted in a reduction of stress for the child? The answer is probably yes. Taylor and O'Connor (1989) found that the stay of children accompanied by a resident parent was 31% shorter than for those whose parents were not resident.

There are still reports that very young children may show a degree of regression following hospital admission – their language becomes more babyish, they may wet the bed at night, they may want to eat with a spoon rather than a fork (see Wanschura & Loschenkohl, 1979). Children who are not well-prepared and are subject to invasive procedures show increased verbal and physical aggression, behavioural regression and greater anxiety. Aisenberg, Wolff, Rosenthal and Nadas (1973) reported that 93% of 4–6 year olds, 71% of 6–12 year olds and 43% of 12–16 year olds were affected in this way.

In contrast, Peterson and Shigetomi (1983) contacted mothers of children one year after admission for routine tonsillectomies, and found that few children showed long-term disturbance. Indeed, the children seemed to view the whole experience rather positively (especially the ice-cream!). Shannon, Ferguson and Dimond (1984) studied a cohort of 1048 New Zealand children, and compared behaviour at 6 years of age, depending on previous hospital experience. They were unable to find evidence of behaviour disturbance and concluded that 'contemporary paediatric inpatient care has little effect on subsequent behaviour'.

It is essential that attempts are made to replicate these findings. While improved paediatric care has undoubtedly reduced the risk of adverse effects for children undergoing occasional or short admissions, the possibility of long-term, serious sequelae remain for some. The risk is greater for those experiencing frequent admissions, and this includes children with chronic disease. Apart from the practical improvements in care, many hospitals now offer a variety of intervention programmes to familiarise children with hospital and treatment, and hopefully reduce associated fear or anxiety.

Preparation for hospital

Very young children are often poorly informed and ill-prepared for what happens in hospital. Recognition of this has resulted in diverse attempts to prepare them in advance. Vernon, Foley, Sipowicz and Schulman (1965) state that preparation should (1) provide information to the child (2) encourage emotional expression and (3) establish a trusting relationship with hospital staff. There has been less theory behind all this than might be considered ideal, and rather more blind enthusiasm. Preparation has been aimed primarily at children about to undergo short-term, routine surgery. Rather less attention has been given to the needs of chronically sick children undergoing repeated and painful procedures. Recently there has been a move to involve parents in the preparation of their children. In addition, it is acknowledged that it is impossible to prepare children admitted for traumatic injury, and to get round this problem, some centres have advocated that healthy children in the community should be informed about what goes on in hospital.

Researchers are not always agreed on what constitutes *success* in terms of preparation. Most commonly, the children's *anxiety* or *fear* has been assessed on standardised assessment scales, with the hope that children exposed to preparation will show a reduction in scores over those not exposed to preparation. Other measures are more *behavioural*. For example, observations of children's behaviour are made on the ward generally, or during painful procedures. It is hoped that preparation is associated with improved (usually more compliant) behaviour. Similarly, outcome may be assessed in terms of the amount of *medication* the children require, or *length of hospital stay*. Finally, assessment is often based on *parental reports* of the child's behaviour on return home.

Preparation of well children

Preparation of well children is the only form of preparation possible for many children, including those admitted following accident or injury, or those admitted suddenly as a result of acute or chronic illness (Peterson & Brownlee-Duffeck, 1984). Programmes aimed at well children may reach large numbers of children and are often highly innovative and well-intentioned. The aim is to inform children about what goes on in hospitals, familiarise them with equipment and standard procedures and, it is generally hoped, reduce anxiety and fear should the need for hospitalisation arise.

The evaluation of these programmes is a daunting task. However large the group prepared, it is not likely that many children will require admission within a reasonably short time of the programme. For this reason, many evaluations rely on post hoc measures of consumer satisfaction, or author impressions.

School-based programmes tend to adopt one of three approaches. Hospital tours may be used, where the emphasis is on familiarising the child with the local hospital. Alternatively, the hospital may come to the child – play hospitals are set up in schools and children given the opportunity to play with equipment. Finally, slide-shows or video-films are used.

Hospital tours have been described by McGarvey (1983). Small groups of children (10), with teachers and some mothers, were introduced to various sides of hospital life. They were allowed to climb into a hospital bed, and encouraged to talk about how it feels to be in a 'bed with rails'. The purpose of the rails (for safety and not punishment) was emphasised. Simple procedures, such as taking oral temperatures and pulses, were demonstrated. Where appropriate, children were sometimes introduced to patients and allowed to discuss their illness and procedures. These tours were reported to be very successful in terms of creating an enjoyable experience of the hospital. Teachers reported that children frequently played 'hospitals' following the visits, and there were no indications that any child found the visit stressful. Follow-up on three children who were subsequently admitted suggested that the hospital tour was useful in enabling the children to adjust readily to hospital life.

Other authors (see Brett, 1983) prefer to set up mini-hospitals in schools. Elkins and Roberts (1984), for example, described a 'pretend hospital'. The following scenes were created: admissions, ward, radiology, surgery and special care. Hospital volunteers dressed up as various personnel (nurse, surgeon, etc.) and described to the children what happens at each of the five scenes. Children who took part in this programme showed fewer medical fears and had improved medical knowledge over those who did not participate.

A similar procedure was adopted by Eiser and Hanson (1989). A miniature hospital was set up in an empty classroom in school. It was divided into four areas.

The *reception* area consisted of a table and two chairs opposite to each other. On the table was a telephone, note-pad and pencil. There was also a display-rack containing a selection of health education leaflets.

The *hospital ward* consisted of two beds made with blankets, and a baby's cot, complete with doll. There was a food table on one of the beds, and a 'drip' hanging at the side. On a small table nearby were several pairs of rubber gloves, cotton face-masks and head-covers (of the type used in surgery). On a series of open shelves was an array of medical equipment, including a stethoscope, syringe, tweezers, respiratory mask and nursing bowls.

In the *X-ray* area was a hard table covered with a sheet. Above the table was a pretend light that could be swung through a semi-circle, and two X-ray pictures were hung on the wall.

In the *surgery* area was another hard table covered by a sheet. There was also another green sheet on top, with a hole through which the 'surgery' could be performed. On nearby shelves were a number of green surgical overalls, hats, masks, gloves and overshoes. In addition, there was a set of surgical equipment, including knives, tweezers, scissors, etc.

There was also a selection of dressing-up clothes. There were nursing uniforms of several grades (dark blue for sister, light blue for staff nurse, green for students), a doctor's white coat and various 'patient' outfits: pyjamas, nighties and dressing-gowns.

The equipment was explained to the children by a school nurse. Ample opportunity for play was allowed. In addition, the children undertook related classroom projects on a range of topics, including health and cleanliness, food and hygiene, birth and reproduction and the dangers of smoking. The project was evaluated by analysis of children's play before and after the teaching sessions. Children showed increased hospital-related knowledge. Perhaps more importantly, in subsequent 'doctors and nurses' play the children showed greater rapport and empathy with patients.

A third method involves the use of videos, films or slide and audiotape presentations. Klinzing and Klinzing (1977) used a video-tape in which a TV personality narrated the hospital experience of a child and puppet model from admission to discharge. A comparison video involving the same TV personality and a non-related hospital experience was also used. Seventy-three children aged between 2 and 5 years watched one or other video. More knowledge and more positive attitudes to hospital were reported among those viewing the hospital video.

Evaluations of well child programmes

Systematic evaluations have been reported by Klinzing and Klinzing (1977), Roberts, Wortele, Boone, Ginther and Elkins (1981), Elkins and Roberts (1985) and Peterson and Ridley-Johnson (1983). The results generally point to intervention techniques resulting in increases in hospital-related knowledge, although there is less con-sistency in terms of successful reduction of anxiety and fear.

It is difficult to conclude categorically that any one method of intervention is superior to another. For one reason, there is no stan-dard content to the programmes, so that comparisons involve not only different methods, but also different concepts and information. Thus, in one study (see Peterson & Ridley-Johnson, 1983) a lecture may be as good as a film in informing children, but changes in the contents of one or the other might result in quite different results.

The lack of impact in terms of reducing anxiety and fear may be the result of a bias in selection of children involved. Both Elkins and Roberts (1985) and Peterson and Ridley-Johnson (1983) report that the level of hospital-related fear in their sample was low prior to intervention. Evaluations of these methods with children who are genuinely fearful are very necessary.

It is not altogether clear, however, at what level these programmes are successful; whether by increasing hospital-related knowledge, reducing anxiety or helping children develop appropriate coping skills. Future work needs to address some of these issues regarding the processes involved in developing children's hospital-related awareness.

Despite these difficulties, education of well children is the only means of informing some children about hospital. For this reason, difficulties in evaluation techniques should not be used as an argument against the continuing development of more effective programmes.

Preparation of acutely sick children

Children undergoing routine surgery are the easiest group to prepare. Their admissions are planned, their treatment and recovery predictable.It is hardly surprising then that much work on preparation has focused on this group. Though there remain unanswered questions about the effectiveness of different types of preparation, about the timing of preparation and about who should be responsible for preparation, a number of major reviews have concluded that *any preparation is better than none* (Goslin, 1978; Eiser, 1985; Elkins & Roberts, 1983; Peterson & Mori, 1988; Rodin, 1983; Lavigne & Burns, 1981).

In the survey by Peterson and Ridley-Johnson (1980) it was found that 70% of American hospitals claimed that they used some form of preparation. The most popular methods included the following: colouring or story books (55%), play therapy (48%), films or videos (37%), puppet shows (21%), relaxation training (16%), and pre-admission tours (27%).

COLOURING OR STORY BOOKS: This constitutes the simplest and cheapest method of preparation, and offers the child a minimal amount of preparation. Booklets and colouring sheets are easily distributed and can be taken up by children whenever they feel interested. Printed drawings of the human body can be used to explain illness and medical treatment. There are also widely available leaflets which are cheap and provide patients with a minimum of information. In addition, there is now a wide selection of books for children of all ages directed generally at the hospital experience or more specifically at individual diseases (Altschuler, 1974; Crocker, 1979).

PLAY THERAPY: Play is an essential part of a child's normal life. Play may simply be seen as an activity to take the child's mind away from a stressful situation, but it provides other functions too. Children play at home and at school, and by providing play facilities in hospital, a continuity is created which serves to reduce the distinctiveness of hospital. Play also enables the child to work through anxieties related to being away from home, or to the treatment. For the child, acting out anxieties is a way of handling them. Finally, directed play enables the child to learn about the hospital experience and procedures. Directed play with a play leader is a means to educate the child about aspects of the treatment, as well as facilitating the expression of anxieties and fears. This kind of preparation is specially suitable for young or less verbal children. Play therapy can be used to give procedural and sensory information (Abbott, Hansen & Lewis, 1970), to clear up misconceptions about surgery (Chan, 1980) or to allow the child to express fear (Crowl, 1980).

Cassell and Paul (1967) studied 40 children aged between 3 and 11 years admitted for cardiac catheterisation. Play therapy was given to half the children. This involved two 30-minute sessions, one before and one following the medical procedures. Puppets depicting the child, nurse and cardiologist and mock-up miniature equipment were given to the child. Initially the therapist took on the role of the cardiologist and in this way the procedure was explained to the child. Then the roles were reversed with the therapist playing the role of patient, and showing particularly that it was legitimate for the patient to cry if treatment hurt. The two groups were then compared by means of parental questionnaires, ward observations and behaviour during procedures. Children who received play therapy showed less emotional disturbance during procedures and expressed a greater willingness to return to hospital. There were however no differences between the groups on parent-rated behaviour when the child returned home.

Play therapy has greatest potential in helping children come to terms with severe illness or disability. There have been a number of case reports involving children undergoing limb amputations, renal disease or open-heart surgery. Few of these studies, however, have systematically evaluated the effects of play therapy. Nevertheless, play therapy sessions provide an opportunity for children to understand and master their treatment which is unequalled by other methods of preparation. Linn, Beardslee and Patenaude (1986), in their study of children undergoing bone-marrow transplants, note that play therapy enables the child to act out anxieties, and come to terms with them by achieving mastery in the role of doctor or nurse. Also, the therapist in the role of patient is able to verbalise feelings of anger, fear or sadness that the child may be unable to express directly. Issues related to the context of play therapy may give an insight into the child's concerns or misunderstandings about treatment that otherwise would remain obscure to nursing staff.

FILMS: Films or videos to prepare children for hospital have been more extensively evaluated than any other preparation technique. Particularly as the number of video-sets available has increased, there has been a rapid growth in development of video-films for children.

Almost without exception, these videos are directed at children suffering relatively minor and short-term illnesses (e.g. tonsillectomies). In fact, the real limitation of this method seems to be that it is not generally suitable for children with serious or chronic illness, since these children do not undergo routine or predictable treatment. You cannot fully prepare children for treatment if you are not sure yourself what will be involved!

However, for children undergoing routine surgery, the method has potential. The content of these videos generally includes details of the hospital setting and wards so that children know what to expect from the environment. In addition, the videos usually follow one particular child through admission, treatment, and discharge. Films typically depict a child, initially fearful of the hospital, cooperating with treatment, and leaving hospital with no ill-effects.

Evaluations of the effectiveness of these videos usually entail a comparison between two groups of children: one who see the hospital film and another who watch a film of similar length and interest value but on a quite different topic. Using such a method, Melamed (1981) reported a reduction in anxiety, post-hospital fears, palmar sweat index, and post-operative complications for children viewing the hospital film. Similar support for this method has been reported by Vernon & Bailey (1974), Ferguson (1979) and many others.

There is no doubt that, if used properly, videos can make an important contribution to preparing children for hospitalisation. The danger comes if the videos are shown to groups of children, with no provision made to answer their questions that arise from the content of the video. There has to be an opportunity for children to voice their anxieties and receive clarification on points that they find confusing. Videos need to be seen as the starting-point of adequate preparation, rather than an end in themselves.

In addition, the content of the films is usually standard across a wide age-range. It would be relatively easy to produce films that addressed the concerns of children of different ages or ethnic backgrounds, but this is not common practice. Yet there seems no foundation for the assumption that informational needs are independent of these variables.

RELAXATION TRAINING AND STRESS INOCULATION: Coping skills training, or cognitive behavioural stress inoculation, is based on the stress-inoculation model developed by Meichenbaum (1975). It has been used in a variety of situations to reduce maladaptive behaviours (Barrios & Shigetomi, 1980; Peterson & Brownlee-

Duffeck, 1984). The processes whereby coping skills may facilitate more appropriate responses are several (Leventhal, 1982; Peterson & Shigetomi, 1981). Coping skills are thought to be associated with increased parental reinforcement for relaxed responding, increased active responding (to reduce fearful interpretation and promote habituation to bodily sensations) and increased perceptions of control. Coping skills training involves a variety of techniques, including deep-muscle relaxation, imagery distraction or self-instruction.

In one of the first reports involving the use of coping skills training with children prior to hospitalisation, Peterson and Shigetomi (1981) divided their sample into four groups. The first group received basic information, given by a puppet model. The second was exposed to the puppet model and a commercial modelling video. The third group received coping skills training and the fourth group received all three interventions. Children who received the coping skills training were rated as less upset and more cooperative by their parents, observers and nurses, both before and after surgery. However, the combination of modelling and coping techniques seemed especially valuable – children who received all three interventions being rated as least upset.

These procedures were extended by Zastowny, Kirschenbaum and Meng (1986). These authors showed children a filmed puppetry informational intervention. In addition, one group also received parent-mediated anxiety reduction (see Skipper, Leonard & Rhymes, 1968). That is, parents learned relaxation and other procedures to help them reduce their own stress. A second group received parent-assisted training in coping skills (Meichenbaum, 1975). In this group, parents learned how to help their children cope with distress.

Thirty-three children aged between 6 and 10 years who were to be admitted for routine elective surgery took part in the study. Compared with children who received 'information only', those in the anxiety-reduction and coping skills groups reported less fearfulness, and their parents also reported fewer maladaptive behaviours during hospitalisation and less problem behaviours immediately before and immediately after hospital admission.

Coping skills training seems to have considerable potential in preparing children for hospitalisation. Zastowny and his colleagues noted that those who received coping skills training were especially adaptive when confronted with painful medical procedures. Since these children learned specific skills to cope with these procedures, it may be that this resulted in an increased perception of control accompanied by decreased levels of physiological arousal and distress. An alternative explanation may be that training produced a cognitive schema about the nature of experience, and this guided them in handling the situation (Leventhal, 1982). Further analysis of the processes whereby improved coping skills are associated with more adaptive responses is necessary.

Regardless of the processes whereby coping skills training is effective, there is evidence that the skills can be generalised to stressful situations outside the hospital setting. According to Peterson and Shigetomi (1982), 33% of their sample successfully used coping skills outside the hospital. If these results are substantiated, it is particularly important to pursue research aimed at developing these techniques.

Some hospitals also use puppet shows and pre-admission tours (described on p. 18) to inform children before admission.

The role of parents

Some parents can feel more tense about their child's admission to hospital than even the child feels. Parents may have memories of a traumatic admission when they were children, or have developed very negative views of hospital staff over the years. They may also be more acutely aware of the potential seriousness of the child's condition, or imagine that the child's illness is more serious than it really is. They may also have many practical problems to cope with, especially in relation to reorganising life at home and work. Arrangements have to be made for other children to be cared for or collected from school, and meals prepared in advance. At work, too, reorganisations need to be made. Parents can also find it difficult just to get to hospital, and this applies particularly when people have to travel long distances to get to major treatment centres. In England, for some parents coming from country districts into London, the final straw may well be having to negotiate one's way round the London underground.

Parents then are fairly stressed, and this is readily communicated to the child. According to van der Veer (1949), the parents' mental state can be transmitted to the child via a process of 'emotional contagion': tense parents have tense children.

Bush, Melamed, Sheras and Greenbaum (1986) observed mothers and their children immediately before examination in a paediatric clinic. Mothers who were highly emotional and appeared agitated, who ignored their child or needed much reassurance from medical staff, had children who were also very distressed. In contrast, mothers who demonstrated a range of coping behaviours (for example, distracting their child with games or reading books) had children who were considerably less distressed. Thus, the presence of a parent was beneficial for some children, but not for others.

These findings, together with work concerned with the value of maternal presence during painful procedures (see Chapter 3), do not suggest that the presence of a parent is necessarily advantageous to the child. The relationship between parent and child during hospitalisation and painful treatments is dependent on a number of factors, including the pre-existing relationship (Robertson, 1958), the parents' family and social supports (Visintainer & Wolfer, 1975) and the parents' reactions to illness and hospitalisation (Roskies, Mongeon & Gagnon-Lefebvre, 1978).

The parental role in shaping the child's response is clearly critical. Where parents give detailed information in response to the child's self-initiated questions, reductions in child anxiety have been documented (Heffernan & Azarnoff, 1971). (However, this was not true for children who did not ask questions. In these cases, minimal information resulted in reduced anxiety.)

If parents can play a major role in reducing their child's anxiety about procedures, it suggests that preparation of parents may provide the key to the most successful preparation of children. Increasingly this view is being recognised. Stress-point preparation for the mother (Skipper, Leonard & Rhymes, 1968) or the mother and child (Wolfer & Visintainer, 1979) appears to be successful. Pinto and Hollandsworth (1984) used parents as an aid in preparation based on modelling videos, and the studies by Zastowny, Kirschenbaum and Meng (1986) and Peterson and Shigetomi (1981) used parents to train children in the use of specific coping strategies. Wherever possible, methods which help parents to understand procedures may prove highly successful, not only by reducing their own anxiety, but also because parents are often in a unique position to relate to, and empathise with, their own child.

Conclusions

It may be felt intuitively that preparing children for hospital is a valuable exercise, but so far a large investment of research effort has failed to demonstrate convincingly the role of preparation in reducing hospital-related stress. A number of techniques have been developed, some being easier to put into practice than others. The real criticism is that the techniques are not always suitable for the children really in need. We know that certain children are more vulnerable, especially younger ones (Goslin, 1978), or those from disadvantaged backgrounds (Quinton & Rutter, 1976). These factors are not taken into account in evaluations. For convenience, we may study older children (since they can verbalise their responses, see Peterson, Schultheis, Ridley-Johnson, Miller & Tracy, 1984) and more socially advantaged groups (because they are more easily available). The potential value of different techniques for children most likely to be distressed by hospital is often not investigated.

A particularly critical review of the literature was made by Saille, Burgmeier and Schmidt (1988). They conducted a meta-analysis of 75 studies concerned with preparing children for hospitalisation and surgery. As a result, it was concluded that 'the mean effect size obtained by psychological preparation – scarcely half a standard deviation – seems to be modest' (p. 124). The authors consequently questioned the effectiveness of preparation techniques. Their review raises difficult questions about methodological techniques and statistical rigour, as well as highlighting areas of evaluation that have been neglected. Together with the review by Peterson and Mori (1988), issues are raised about the discrepancies between what actually happens in hospitals, and the focus of research questions and activities. There is a real need to disseminate research findings to practitioners. Otherwise there is little relationship between the clinical practice of preparation and the research literature.

Already it is apparent that hospitals do not use well-researched techniques, such as filmed modelling, coping or play therapy, to prepare children. Instead, they rely on hospital tours, or verbal descriptions of treatment, which have received little research attention. The gap between hospital practice and research interests is very wide indeed.

In the past, attempts to prepare children have been made by psychologists, teachers or nurses. There has not always been cooperation between these groups, and little successful communication of findings to parents or medical staff. There remains a continuing need to develop, improve and make available preparation techniques for all hospitalised children.

3

The nature of pain

Introduction

Pain is a very individual experience. Many 'painful' incidents which occur to young children (like falling off their bike or grazing an elbow) can be relieved easily by a kiss, bar of chocolate or bag of crisps! Perhaps the ease with which children are comforted in this way makes it difficult for us to appreciate the child's feelings in more serious circumstances.

Regardless of the 'objective' intensity of any pain stimulus, individuals vary enormously in their responses. Some people appear to experience a great deal of pain, yet remain cheerful, optimistic and good company. Others make much more fuss: they like to discuss their pain and perhaps make us feel so guilty or uncomfortable that we begin to avoid their company. It is very difficult for a healthy individual to imagine what it is like to live with chronic pain. Pain is invisible; we have to rely on people's reports of their pain – perhaps they exaggerate a little?

The knowledge that a child is in severe pain, and that there is nothing that can really be done to relieve it, is very distressing for the family, and also for medical staff. Yet extreme pain is a routine part of life for many children with conditions such as leukaemia or haemophilia, as well as for those treated for burns. In all these cases, treatment entails frequent and highly distressing procedures.

Traditionally, little attention was paid to issues of childhood pain. It was even argued that young children did not experience pain, at least, not as acutely as adults. Physiological differences in myelination and pain thresholds were thought to account for these effects. This position is now challenged from a variety of viewpoints. Changes in pain thresholds and tolerance certainly occur throughout childhood, but it is clear that infants experience pain sensations from birth.

McGrath and Unruh (1987) argued that the myth that infants do not learn from past painful experiences contributes to the tendency to undermedicate infants. Certainly, there is considerable evidence that children and adults with the same diagnoses are treated differently in terms of analgesic medication. Schechter, Allen and Hanson (1986) compared 90 children with 90 adults in four diagnostic categories (hernias, appendectomies, burns and fractured femurs). On average, adults received 2.2 doses of narcotics per day, while children received 1.1. The difference between adults and children increased with the length of hospital stay. This raises the question that medical staff may be less inclined to recognise discomfort and pain in children compared with adults.

The measurement and assessment of pain

The International Association for the Study of Pain has defined pain as follows:

> An unpleasant sensory and emotional experience associated with actual or potential tissue damage or described in terms of damage.
> (Merskey, 1986, p. S217)

Pain is undoubtedly a subjective experience; it can be measured only in terms of (1) what people report about their experiences (self-report methods); (2) how they behave in response to pain (behavioural methods); or (3) how their bodies react to pain (physiological methods) (McGrath & Unruh, 1987). While the measurement and assessment of pain is difficult in adults, it poses even greater problems with regard to children.

> With children, the problems of pain measurement and assessment are confounded: by children's constantly developing but relatively limited cognitive ability to understand what is being asked of them in pain measurement; by children's limited verbal skills, by our lack of understanding of the developing nervous system and its influence on pain perception in children; by the usually limited experience children have had of pain; by the limited behavioral competencies that children (especially very young children) have, and, finally, by the lack of research and or subsequent limited understanding of children's pain behavior and the physiology of pain in children.
> (McGrath & Unruh, 1987, p. 74)

Distinctions between measurement and assessment

The measurement of any concept normally involves the application of some metric to a specific component. With respect to pain, intensity is usually measured. The assessment of pain covers a much broader perspective, and attempts to account for differences in the affective response to a stimulus, the role of family styles on perception of pain, the impact on families of having a child in pain, and the meaning of pain to the child and family. While some progress has been made in developing measures of intensity of pain, there have so far been few attempts to assess subjective aspects of pain in a standardised way.

Measurement of pain

Pain has a number of different components and this is reflected in the range of instruments developed to measure pain. Researchers are not always in agreeement as to the best way to conceptualise the different components of pain. Melzack (1983) suggested that pain could be divided into 'pain sensations' and reactions to pain. McGrath and his colleagues (McGrath & Unruh, 1987) favour a distinction that takes into account (1) the cognitive or self-report; (2) the behaviour; and (3) the physiological components.

Cognitive or self-report methods

Clinicians often rely on simple questions, such as 'How is your pain today?', to assess children's pain. Clearly, however, responses to such questions may be influenced by many factors, including verbal ability, self-confidence, family variables and preparedness to report symptoms. There is no standard against which to assess the child's response, and retrospective reports of pain are notoriously open to much bias (Ross & Ross, 1984a; Andrasik, Burke, Attanasio & Rosenblum, 1985).

Numerical scales have been developed by Hester (1979) and Richardson, McGrath, Cunningham and Humphreys (1983). In these scales, children are asked to rate their pain on six-point scales (Richardson, McGrath, Cunningham & Humphreys, 1983). These responses correlate well with diary reports of behavioural and subjective components. There is also good inter-rater reliability between parent and child.

A number of investigators have used 'faces scales' (McGrath,

Johnson, Goodman, Schillinger, Dunn & Chapman, 1985). Five to seven faces depicting different degrees of pain are used, and children asked to select the face corresponding to their own pain. These scales are appealing, inexpensive, easy to use with very young children and have good measurement characteristics. The recent proliferation of faces scales has unfortunately not resulted in any generally accepted version (Beyer, 1984).

Visual analogue scales where children indicate their pain on a line, anchored usually at one end by 'no pain' and at the other by 'severe pain' (Abu-Saad, 1984) can be used by children aged 7 years or above. A variant on these, pain thermometers, are also popular (Katz, Kellerman & Siegel, 1980).

A major problem with all self-report measures is that children's responses are swayed considerably by demand characteristics of the situation, and the way in which the question is phrased. Ross and Ross (1984a) for example showed that children described their pain differently to doctors, their mothers or school-friends. A second problem is that young children may lack the cognitive skills to understand or respond to the question in a meaningful way.

Behavioural methods

The most obvious pain behaviour in children that can be measured is crying (Williamson & Williamson, 1983). Other workers have developed categorisations of facial expression in response to pain (Grunau & Craig, 1987).

Behaviour rating scales have also been developed (Craig, McMahon, Morison & Zaskow, 1984; McGrath *et al.*, 1985). A specific scale for use with children undergoing bone-marrow aspirations in cancer treatment was developed by Katz, Kellerman & Siegel (1980). This consists of 13 behavioural items which distinguish between children who can cope well with the procedures (as assessed by nurses' ratings) and those who cope less well. This scale was further modified by Jay and Elliott (1984). The Observation Scale of Behavioural Distress (OSBD) is an 11-item scale which includes provision for (1) continuous behavioural recording in 15 second intervals and (2) a weighting score of severity of distress for each behavioural category in the scale (see Table 3.1). Elliott, Jay and Woody (1987) reported that scores on this scale correlated well with measures of fear, anticipated pain, heart rate and blood pressure, as well as nurses' ratings. However, scores did not correlate with self-reports of experienced pain, perhaps suggesting that

Table 3.1. *Behavioural definitions of categories for the observation scale of behavioural distress*

Category	Definition	Examples
Information seeking	Any questions regarding medical procedure	'Is the needle in?'
Cry	Onset of tears and/or low-pitched nonword sounds of more than 1-second duration	
Scream	Loud, nonword, shrill vocal expressions at high pitch intensity	
Physical restraint	Child is physically restrained with noticeable pressure and/or child is exerting bodily force and resistance in response to restraint	
Verbal resistance	Any intelligible verbal expression of delay, termination or resistance	'Stop' 'I don't want it'
Seeks emotional support	Verbal or nonverbal solicitation of hugs, physical or verbal comfort from parents or staff	'Mama, help me' Pleading to be held
Verbal pain	Any words, phrases or statements in any tense which refer to pain or discomfort	'Ouch' 'My leg hurts' 'That hurt'
Flail	Random gross movements of arms, legs or whole body	Kicking legs; pounding fists
Verbal fear	Any intelligible verbal expressions of fear or apprehension	'I'm scared'
Muscular rigidity	Noticeable contraction of observable body part	Clenched fists; gritted teeth; facial contortions Legs bent tightly upward off radiotherapy table
Nervous behaviour	Physical manifestations of anxiety or fear; consist of repeated, small physical actions	Nail biting; lip chewing

Reprinted from Elliott, Jay and Woody (1987).

the measure is a better indicator of overall anxiety than subjective pain experience.

Behavioural methods of pain assessment are excellent for use with very young children. However, they require well-trained observers and are therefore not useful in all situations.

Physiological methods

Physiological indices associated with pain and anxiety include heart rate (Johnston & Strada, 1986), respiration rate (Williamson & Williamson, 1983; Field & Goldson, 1984), emotional sweating (Harpin & Rutter, 1982), transcutaneous pO_2 (Williamson & Williamson, 1983), pulse and blood pressure (Jay, Elliott, Katz & Siegel, 1984). Early research using physiological measures was based on a unidimensional theory of arousal (Duffy, 1962). However, it is unlikely that any single measure is ever entirely appropriate, and further that complex patterns of autonomic responses are elicited by specific stressors (Lacey, 1967). Multiple, rather than single, measures of physiological arousal are therefore necessary.

Simple physiological measures (such as pulse or blood pressure) appear to be precise and concrete, and may therefore appeal to researchers searching for 'objective' measures. However, individuals may vary substantially in the degree of physiological response to pain. More complex physiological measures, such as sweating, require more complicated equipment than is often readily available (Barrios, Hartman & Shigetomi, 1981).

Assessment of pain

While intensity of pain is clearly an important component of any assessment, many other factors contribute toward an individual's subjective experience of pain. Attempts to assess the influence of these variables have been modelled on the work of Melzack (1975) with adults (Savedra, Gibbons, Tesler, Ward & Wegner, 1982; Tesler, Ward, Savedra, Wegner & Gibbons, 1983).

For example, a questionnaire developed by Tesler *et al.* (1983) included eight questions. Children were asked to describe three events that caused pain, circle the words that described the pain from a list of 24, report on the colour of their pain, select how they felt from a list of 13 possibilities, describe their worst pain, what helps when in pain, and mark on an outline diagram where the pain occurred. This questionnaire has been used with children aged between 9 and 12 years, and differences between the reports of hospitalised and non-hospitalised children have been reported.

McGrath *et al.* (1985) attempted to assess the duration, frequency and location of pain. Children were asked to describe the quality of pain. Intensity of pain was assessed using visual analogue scales, and children were also asked to describe their emotions and expectations about relief of pain. Facial scales were used to assess how children felt about different experiences, both painful (tooth-ache, being smacked) and non-painful (being teased).

Developmental changes in understanding and experience of pain

The way in which a child experiences pain is mediated by a number of factors, not least the attitudes of family and culture. Some parents feel that children should stay home from school if they are slightly under-the-weather; others take a very much more stoic attitude. Perhaps also the age of the child is important; in uncertainty it is more likely that younger children will be allowed to stay at home than older ones. Developmental changes also occur in children's memory for painful experiences (McGrath & Unruh, 1987), their definitions of and understanding of the causes and implications of pain (Ross & Ross, 1984a; Gaffney & Dunn, 1986; 1987), ability to report symptoms (Lewis & Lewis, 1982; Mechanic, 1980; 1983) and availability of appropriate and effective coping strategies (Brown, O'Keeffe, Sanders & Baker, 1986).

Definitions and understanding of pain

Three major studies have investigated children's concepts of pain. Although similar methodological procedures were adopted, different conclusions were drawn.

In the first study, Ross and Ross (1984a) interviewed 994 children aged between 5 and 12 years. Children were asked to define what they meant by pain, describe different causes of pain and explain the potential purpose of pain as a warning signal. There were no age or gender differences in children's reports. Ross and Ross (1984a) specifically noted that it was not possible to categorise children's responses in terms of Piaget's three stages of cognitive development. This is one of the few studies concerned with children's beliefs about health or illness concepts which has not reported that beliefs progress through a series of stages. The appropriateness of a stage model to account for children's beliefs about these issues is discussed in Chapter 6.

In line with much other work, Gaffney and Dunn (1987) concluded that definitions of pain could be accounted for by a stage theory of development. 680 children aged between 5 and 14 years were interviewed about definitions, causes, effects, cures, descriptions and locations of pain. Children described the cause of pain in relation to: (1) illness or disease; (2) malfunction of a body part; (3) trauma; (4) transgression involving eating; (5) transgression involving other activities; (6) transgression of adult rules; (7) health risk behaviours (smoking); (8) transgressions implicating punishment; (9) psychological factors; (10) need states (hunger); (11) physiological explanations (pain as a warning); and (12) contamination (by germs).

Almost half of the children felt that transgressions of one kind or another were involved in causing pain. The second major finding of this study was the increase with age in use of objective and abstract explanations of pain.

Gaffney and Dunn (1986) also reported (using the same sample of children) that definitions of pain could be categorised in one of the three stages of cognitive development described by Piaget. In the pre-operational age-group, children attended to essentially 'perceptual' features of a painful experience; i.e. pain was defined in terms of location, or something that hurts. They did not understand that pain might indicate something more serious. During the concrete-operational stage, children began to use more abstract generalisations, were capable of forming analogies or mentioned the psychological effects of pain. Pain was something inside them, rather than restricted to a specific location. Finally, in the formal operational stage, children were able to define pain in physical, psychological or psychosocial terms. Despite this categorisation, Gaffney and Dunn (1986) had some reservations about their stage account. They also noted that there were no sudden developments in children's definitions of pain, and that definitions typical of less mature stages could co-exist with more mature explanations.

Taken together, these studies suggest a wide variability in understanding of pain at all ages. The work is subject to similar criticisms as have been levelled at other attempts to trace developmental changes in children's concepts of health or illness (Burbach & Peterson, 1986; Eiser, 1989). Physicians often rely on parents' reports of a child's pain experience (Barr, 1983). The work by Ross and Ross (1984a) and Gaffney and Dunn (1986; 1987) suggests that children are able to verbalise their feelings and understanding of the cause of pain. However, in all these studies, responses were elicited from healthy children, with little, if any, experience of severe or chronic pain. Parallel research involving children who have had some experience of pain is necessary to understand the influence of experience on verbal reports of pain. Attention to children's idiosyncratic beliefs should become an integral part of assessment procedures and form the basis on which appropriate intervention is developed.

Symptom-reporting

The extent to which we can understand an individual's subjective experience of pain is affected by the frequency with which symptoms are reported. Some individuals report symptoms at the first sign of distress; others only report symptoms when severe distress is experienced. It is generally assumed that the predisposition to report pain symptoms is part of a wider personality trait rather than specific to a particular symptom. Gochman (1971), for example, found that children who felt vulnerable and reported that they had little control over their lives were more likely to report symptoms and utilise medical services.

Lewis and Lewis (1982) found that a very small percentage (8–12%) of children made over half the visits to a school health service (children were encouraged to initiate their own visits to the service). Girls, first-borns and children of lower social class were the highest users. In a 16-year follow-up involving 350 mother–child pairs, Mechanic (1980; 1983) found that the best predictors of the child's symptom-reporting were the number of family problems reported by the mother, her own symptoms, the number of days of school missed by the child and the teacher's perception of the child's stoicism. Mechanic and Hansell (1987) found that self-assessments of health in adolescents were not related to illness experience, but to feelings of well-being, competence and participation in sports and exercise. Physical symptoms tended to be associated with depression and lower self-esteem. Miller (1987) presented extensive evidence to suggest that individuals differ in the extent to which they notice symptoms, the severity of symptoms experienced immediately before they seek medical advice, and the extent to which they report that treatment is successful in reducing symptoms. It would appear that there are large individual differences in symptom-reporting which can influence when professional advice is sought, and how effective treatment is perceived to be.

Coping strategies

Before discussing some of the interventions that have been developed to help children manage pain experiences, it is worth noting the extent to which they use self-initiated coping strategies spontaneously. Ross and Ross (1984a) found that 213 of their sample of 994 children used self-initiated coping strategies. The most frequently used methods included distraction and physical activity (such as clenching the fist or pinching the skin), with a small proportion reporting the use of thought-stopping, relaxation or imagery and fantasising. Others had apparently not developed any strategies to deal with pain.

Brown, O'Keeffe, Sanders and Baker (1986) also suggest that many children do not intuitively adopt coping strategies. One hundred children at each of five age-levels (8–9, 10–11, 12–13, 14–15 and 16–18 years) were interviewed. The children were asked to describe their feelings associated with (a) a visit to the dentist, (b) presenting a report to the class, and (c) a situation of their own choosing that 'has worried you recently'. The number of children reporting the use of any kind of coping strategy increased with age. The most frequently described strategy at all ages involved 'positive self-talk'. With increasing age, children reported a greater number of potential strategies that they might use. However, a relatively large number of children failed to report any coping strategies at all (64% of the total sample).

In contrast, Band and Weisz (1988) concluded that in a variety of stressful situations, children did report using self-initiated coping strategies. Children of 6, 9 and 12 years were asked to recall stressful episodes involving six different situations (separation, medical stress, school failure, a time when your mum or dad was mad at you, a time when another child said something mean and a time when you had an accident and got hurt). Children were asked to describe what happened, report how they felt and all that they had done to handle the situation. Responses were coded in terms of primary or secondary coping or relinquished control. (Primary coping was defined in terms of efforts to influence objective events and secondary coping as efforts aimed at maximising one's goodness-of-fit with conditions as they are. This approach is often seen to be complementary with the problem/emotion-focused model.)

Most children reported that they actively tried to handle stressful situations; only 3.5% of the total number of responses were coded as relinquished control. However, preferred styles of coping varied across situations with school failure eliciting high levels of primary coping and medical stress eliciting high levels of secondary coping. Styles also differed with age. Older children reported a decrease in preference for primary coping and increase in secondary coping, especially in relation to stressful medication procedures. Band and

Weisz (1988) concluded that children make very positive efforts to cope with everyday stresses, and that these efforts are influenced both by situational constraints and cognitive development.

Research concerned with chronically sick patients needs to be integrated with research describing developmental changes in normal coping behaviour, so that the responses of the chronically sick child are seen to reflect normal development, rather than be categorised as deviant and maladaptive. The counselling and interventions offered to these patients can then also be phrased within this general developmental framework.

These studies provide important data about the range of coping strategies children potentially have available. Clearly, however, the strategies children report that they might use may differ substantially from those that are actually used in any crisis situation. Nevertheless, the findings concerning the changes in coping strategies used by healthy children of different ages may have important implications for understanding behaviour in stressful medical situations, and for developing appropriate interventions.

Intervention strategies

Intervention strategies have usually been developed with one of four aims. Treatments may focus on attempts to change (1) pain behaviour; (2) family context and reactions to pain behaviour; (3) the child's imagination, attention or thinking; or (4) physiological responses.

Relaxation

Relaxation is an essential component of most forms of pain therapy, and works by decreasing the activity of the sympathetic and motor nervous systems. Techniques may often involve 'progressive relaxation', where patients are taught to relax individual muscle groups. The method is cheap and appropriate for a wide range of pain control.

Puppet therapy

Puppet therapy has been used both to explain medical procedures to children and to encourage feelings of control and mastery during the procedure itself (Cassell, 1965; Linn, 1978). The procedure has also been used with children undergoing bone-marrow aspirations.

Linn, Beardslee and Patenaude (1986) used animal puppets in a series of sessions primarily to develop the child's sense of mastery. Children were able to express feelings via the puppets, and could use the puppets to act out their own feelings, or their perceptions of the roles of doctor, parent and others. In the work by Linn *et al.*, sessions focused particularly on themes around medical procedures, body integrity, confinement, abandonment and the expressions of rage and fear. The method is hoped to provide access to aspects of children's anxiety that are not always addressed in conventional dialogue.

Hypnosis

Hypnosis is not well-defined, and not always distinguishable from other techniques such as imagery (Olness, 1981), imaginative involvement (Kuttner, 1984) or distraction. Formal hypnotic techniques are rarely used with preadolescent children, although those involving fantasy or dissociation are popular. The exact procedures that authors adopt in interventions are not always clear, and distinctions between techniques defined as hypnosis in some studies and distractions or imagery in others are often cloudy.

Nevertheless 'hypnosis' is a popular technique (LeBaron & Hilgard, 1984), especially for children undergoing bone-marrow aspirations (BMAs) or other treatments used in the care of leukaemia patients (Hilgard & LeBaron, 1982; Ellenberg, Kellerman, Dash, Higgins & Zeltzer, 1980; Olness, 1981; Zeltzer, 1980). Most studies concentrate on children aged 6 years and above, and there is some debate as to the efficacy of hypnotic procedures used with children below this age (Hilgard & Morgan, 1976).

While many reports are based on clinical case studies, or lack objective measures of distress, two studies in particular report fairly rigorous evaluations. Zeltzer and LeBaron (1982) compared hypnosis with supportive counselling combined with distraction in reducing distress among 33 cancer patients (aged 6–17 years). The hypnosis intervention consisted of an individual programme of imagery and fantasy. Children were told exciting or funny stories and then asked questions to stimulate the imagination. Deep-breathing instructions were combined with the imagery techniques. These techniques were compared with distraction at practice sessions to decrease fear. (For example, children were encouraged to focus attention on objects in the room rather than to fantasise.)

Both techniques were of help to some patients, although hypnosis was concluded to be the superior technique for a greater number of patients. Zeltzer and LeBaron (1982) felt that children were able to focus attention for longer in the imagery condition, compared with focusing on concrete objects in the room.

A variant on this procedure was reported by Kuttner (1984). Again, hypnosis was compared with distraction, and in addition a control group who received no intervention was included. Both treatment groups reported less anxiety than the control group, although the hypnosis group reported the least. There were no effects of either treatment on children's self-reports of pain. Younger children appeared to be helped significantly more by the hypnotic techniques than older children.

Coping and stress-inoculation

These techniques are similar to those developed to help children cope with hospitalisation decribed in the previous chapter. Children are first provided with information about the stressor, then taught a number of coping techniques, and finally given the opportunity to practice the coping skills during exposure to relevant stressors.

This approach was developed by Jay, Elliott, Ozolins, Olson and Pruitt (1985) for children undergoing bone-marrow aspirations (BMAs). There are five components to the procedure. Children are first shown a video film in which another child is undergoing a BMA. The child describes her feelings throughout the procedure and models positive coping behaviour. The model expresses anxiety but also demonstrates successful coping and mastery. Following the film, children are taught simple breathing exercises to be used to detract attention from the procedure. Children are also given positive reinforcement in the form of a small trophy as a 'symbol of mastery and courage'. The idea of the trophy is to encourage children to view the simulation as a challenge. Help is provided to enable them to meet the challenge and therefore it is hoped that they will be able to maintain self-esteem and self-worth by facing the challenge.

Emotive imagery involves determining a child's superhero and weaving these images round the medical situation. These images may transform the meaning of pain to the child as well as providing a simple distraction. Finally, children are given dolls and medical kits and allowed to rehearse the procedures. With a doll as patient, the child is given additional information about equipment and procedures. Then the child plays 'patient' and is reminded of the breathing exercises and distraction techniques. Jay, Elliott, Katz and Siegel (*in press*) report considerable success with these procedures.

Conclusions

For children suffering from chronic conditions, especially those with cancer or being treated for burns, invasive medical procedures can be extremely painful and distressing. Unfortunately, for many children, the treatments may continue for many years, and may not be associated with ultimate cure. Many children respond by behaving badly, refusing to cooperate with medical staff, and creating a highly stressful situation for themselves, other patients and medical staff. Other children develop 'anticipatory nausea' and may vomit even before procedures begin.

While some children work out their own ways of coping with these stresses, many do not. A variety of methods have been developed to encourage children to adopt coping skills which will reduce anxiety and fear associated with invasive procedures. There is a continuing need for more systematic evaluation of these procedures, particularly in relation to different treatments and in terms of relative suitabilities for different patients. Age, coping style, previous experience or family support may well influence the degree to which patients are receptive to different interventions. To date, far greater attention has been paid to developing interventions for use with children with cancer undergoing bone-marrow aspirations than for those undergoing other painful treatments.

Although there has been a dramatic increase in the number of instruments developed to measure children's pain, there is little agreement between researchers about the relative merits of different approaches, nor any real move toward an agreed standardised instrument and procedure. Little headway has been made in measuring different components of pain, apart from intensity. New measures are needed that are appropriate for use with infants, and mentally retarded or physically handicapped children.

4

Adjustment in the child with chronic disease

Introduction

At the beginning of this century, children suffered from a wide range of threatening conditions, for which there was rarely any satisfactory medical treatment. This situation has now changed dramatically. Improved sanitation, housing and diet have led to much better general health and resistance to disease. Widespread introduction of vaccination programmes has virtually eradicated conditions like polio, TB or smallpox, and substantially reduced the incidence of measles or whooping cough. Improved neonatal care has reduced the incidence of birth handicaps.

At the same time, there have been enormous strides in the treatment of potentially fatal diseases of childhood. The discovery of insulin in the 1920s has resulted in an effectively normal life-expectancy for diabetics. Antibiotics have greatly increased survival for children with cystic fibrosis, and irradiation and anti-leukaemia drugs have resulted in similarly dramatic chances of survival for children with leukaemia. As a result, a great deal of the work-load for paediatricians today centres on the care of children with these 'chronic diseases'. These conditions affect children for a period of at least 3 months, but typically for life. They cannot be cured. Instead, treatment is aimed at helping children become responsible for as much of the treatment as possible, in order to foster some independence from parents and the medical profession. In addition, treatment is aimed at reducing the potentially negative effects of the condition as far as possible, and enabling the child to adopt a normal life-style.

Some 10–12% of children suffer from chronic disease (Hobbs & Perrin, 1985; Cadman, Boyle, Szatmari & Offord, 1987). The most common is asthma. The incidence of other diseases is shown in Table 1.1.

Caring for a chronically sick child is extremely demanding both physically and emotionally. Parents are taught to undertake much of the routine care. They must ensure that appropriate medication is taken. Some diseases (e.g. phenylketonuria, coeliac disease, diabetes, some asthmas) require that children eat restricted diets. These may involve the family making substantial changes in their own eating-habits, and sometimes create difficulties for families in ensuring that the child does eat appropriately. Many rifts occur between children with diabetes and their families over foods children traditionally like to eat (chocolate, fruit squashes, crisps, etc.) but which are banned in the diabetic diet.

Other diseases require parents to learn specific tasks. Children with cystic fibrosis, for example, may require daily physiotherapy, which can be time-consuming and physically exhausting, especially as children become heavier. Those with diabetes need daily tests of blood glucose levels and injections of insulin. Again, these tasks are time-consuming, and require families to learn the specific skills. Many of the routine tasks involved in child-care or domestic work become more demanding, even if they do not require the learning of new skills. Children with asthma, for example, may be allergic to dust. Extra vigilance is therefore needed with domestic chores. Special materials may be required and meticulous cleaning of the child's room is necessary to reduce dust.

The emotional problems for families are no less daunting. Parents must come to terms with the fact that the ambitions they had for the child may never materialise. Illness can compromise achievement by limiting experience and the acquisition of skills. Many diseases are associated with periods of stability followed by periods of relapse and illness (e.g. arthritis, haemophilia or leukaemia). Even when the child is well, families may feel uneasy and anxious that the child will relapse. Other conditions (e.g. muscular dystrophy) result in pro-gressive deterioration, although the exact course and timing of the deterioration is not always predictable. Either way, parents have to cope with a great deal of uncertainty about the child's health and future (Eiser, 1987).

The way in which the family handles these difficulties is likely to determine the child's response to the disease (Burr, 1985; Hauser, Jacobson, Wertlieb, Brink & Wentworth, 1985; Wertlieb, Hauser & Jacobson, 1986; Blotcky, Raczynski, Gurwich & Smith, 1985). For the child, chronic disease may be particularly important in compromising school achievement and academic success. Repeated absences and periods of ill-health can naturally limit achievements. Absences can also interrupt social relationships. In addition, changes in physical appearance can result in children with chronic disease being rejected by peers and becoming unpopular figures in school (e.g. steroids used in the treatment of leukaemia are associated with hair-loss and weight-gain). Restrictions imposed by treatment schedules can be especially difficult for adolescents, resulting in limited social and emotional lives.

The ease with which it is possible to point to all these difficulties has traditionally been taken to imply that children and their families will show a range of behavioural and emotional problems. For this reason, a great deal of research has been concerned to identify the incidence and importance of 'maladjustment' in children with chronic disease. Much of this work is based on the assumption that chronic disease results in general, rather than specific, deficits in adjustment.

It is clear that some children with chronic disease show an increased risk of maladjustment, but many children show no measurable deficits. Recent work therefore has shifted in focus and is now more concerned to identify the coping strategies used by children who manage chronic disease most effectively. Past research has focused on the negative effects of disease to such an extent that the resilience shown by many children and their families has not been recognised. The empirical work in this chapter is concerned exclusively with the incidence of adjustment and maladjustment in children. Adjustment and coping shown by the family will be considered in the following chapter.

The incidence of 'maladjustment' in chronically sick children

Problems of definition

While many researchers have considered problems of 'adjustment' in children with chronic disease, few have attempted to specify exactly what they mean. Concepts of 'adjustment', 'adaptation', 'coping', 'stress', 'competence' and 'dysfunction' are used interchangeably (Rutter, 1981; Compas, 1987; Perrin, Ramsey & Sandler, 1987).

Some detailed discussion of this issue can be found in Pless and Pinkerton (1975). They distinguished two ways in which 'adjustment' is generally used. On the one hand, it can be taken to indicate the extent to which the child functions in everyday life. In this context, school attendance or attainments are often used. Yet chronic disease is almost inevitably associated with interruptions in schooling and subsequently poor achievement, and for this reason these variables are not necessarily good indicators of adjustment. The extent to which we can at all expect children with chronic disease to be indistinguishable from healthy children on these measures is perhaps debatable.

An alternative approach is to measure adjustment in relation to sick-role behaviour. For example, children who comply with medical instructions may be assumed to be better adjusted than those who refuse to cooperate or fail to take prescribed medication. In this case there are no comparable measures available for healthy children.

Pless and Pinkerton (1975) argue that a further definition of the term relates to the *process* of adjustment to the disease. Behind this definition is the idea that there are 'healthy' and 'unhealthy' processes of adjustment or acceptance of the disease. The distinction between 'healthy' and 'unhealthy' adjustment may be of degree rather than of qualitative difference. For example, some denial is often assumed to be healthy, in enabling a child to attempt to cope with difficult situations rather than feel defeated and helpless. Greater degrees of denial, however, may be unhealthy, in that children might attempt tasks that were beyond their capabilities, thereby exposing themselves to physical danger or the risk of depression and loss of self-esteem.

More recent definitions of adjustment focus much more on the notion of competence and coping in specific situations. Hops (1983) defines competence as 'a summary term which reflects social judgement about the general quality of an individual's performance in a given situation'. Many authors opt out of defining what they mean by 'adjustment'. Instead, and increasingly, the term is defined operationally, i.e. as a score on standardised tests.

Methodological issues

Population-based studies are often considered preferable to clinic-based ones (Starfield, 1985), especially since they are more likely to be based on representative samples and the data therefore widely generalisable. Despite this, most research is based on small, often specially selected clinic-samples. No attention is paid to differences between clinics in terms of characteristics of their populations or approaches to care and management. Control groups are not always included, and even where they are, insufficient attention is often paid to relevant variables (Lemanek, Moore, Gresham, Williamson & Kelley, 1986). Most researchers have tried to predict adjustment by investigating the role of specific physical parameters of the disease (e.g. severity) and without taking account of other disease or psychosocial and environmental factors. In the absence of any comprehensive theoretical framework, there is little indication that any factors play a more important role in determining adjustment than any other. Psychiatric interviews and symptom-reports are being replaced by assessments of behaviour (Achenbach & Edelbrook, 1983), self-concept (Piers, 1969) or depression (Kovacs, 1981; Birleson, Hudson, Buchanan & Wolff, 1987) for example. Teacher reports of behaviour, school absence and achievement are also popular (Mearig, 1985). Other standardised measures of competence (Harter, 1981), self-esteem (Lipsitt, 1958), and locus of control (Nowicki & Strickland, 1973) are used.

Theoretical approaches

According to Lipowski (1971), determinants of adjustment are related to three factors: (a) intrapersonal; (b) disease-related, and (c) environmental.

Intrapersonal factors include the child's premorbid personality, intelligence and social background. *Disease-related* factors refer to characteristics of the disease, including the extent to which it is life-threatening, restrictive, chronic, severe, visible, etc. *Environmental* factors include the attitudes of parents, relatives, friends and others to the disease and their perceptions of its implications.

Pless and Pinkerton (1975) proposed an integrated model of adjustment based on these variables. Their basic premise is that adjustment is a dynamic process, continuing from childhood through adult life. Current functioning influences the responses of others, which in turn affects future functioning. At any given time, adjustment reflects the net product of earlier cycles, and is influenced by family attitudes, other social factors, the child's own attributes and response to illness. A series of feed-back loops is set up. For example, genetic and family factors determine attributes of the child (temperament, personality or intelligence). In turn, these child attributes determine self-concept and coping style, and subsequently may influence the way in which others respond.

In practice, research work has tended to concentrate on the influence of one set of variables on the child's adjustment, rather than look at the viability of the model as a whole. In the review of empirical work which follows, it is clear that this approach has yielded a great deal of inconsistent results. There is little evidence, even, that disease parameters (such as severity or chronicity) exert a simple effect on adjustment. Undoubtedly, adjustment is a multi-faceted concept.

It is relatively simple to list variables that might influence adjustment. It is far more difficult to predict how the variables interact to determine the way in which a child responds to illness at any given time. Some attempts to do this have been reported by Wallander and his colleagues (see Varni & Wallander, 1988).

According to Wallander, a set of intrapersonal, interpersonal and social-ecological factors can be defined. *Intrapersonal* factors include the severity of the handicap, and functional independence, as well as personality factors such as temperament or coping style. *Interpersonal factors* include temperament and coping style of the mother, since there is evidence that child and maternal temperament are related to maternal perceptions of role restrictions (Breslau, Staruch & Mortimer, 1982).

Finally, *socio-ecological* factors include marital and family functioning, socioeconomic status, family size and service utilisation. The focus of the model is on the potentially reciprocal nature of these relationships.

So far, the model does not differ very remarkably from that of Pless and Pinkerton (1975), except in details of the components of the three major sets of variables thought to determine adjustment. However, Varni and Wallander (1988) go on to suggest that the reason why families with a chronically sick child are at greater risk of maladjustment relates to the increased number of stressful situations to which they are exposed. 'Stress' is viewed 'as the occurrence of problematic situations requiring a solution or some decision-making process for appropriate action' (Varni & Wallander, 1988, p. 215). A taxonomy of problematic situations for any chronic disease needs to be defined.

If stress is understood in terms of a series of problematic situations or stressors, it follows that an individual's adjustment should be determined in part by their competence in dealing with the situations. 'Competence is defined in terms of the effectiveness of the coping responses emitted when an individual is confronted with problematic situations' (Varni & Wallander, 1988, p. 215). Effective, active coping responses result in a change so that the situation is no longer problematic, while at the same time producing a maximum of additional positive consequences.

For example, a stressor in raising a child with severely handicapping spina bifida may be in the restrictions it puts on the mother who must dress and clean the child daily and, as a result, may exhaust her physical strength and find it necessary to set aside career aspirations. An effective coping response in this problematic situation may be for the mother to learn, through professional consultation, how to teach the child self-care skills. She would thereby increase her competence in dealing with this specific stress of raising a handicapped child. Another example would be a hemophilic adolescent who desires to participate in sports like many of his age-mates, but becomes distraught when he is forbidden by his parents to play basketball. His self-perception may suffer, and he may feel resentful towards his parents. An effective coping response for him might be to consider alternative sports such as swimming or archery as a way of dealing competently with a problematic situation resulting from his disorder.

(Varni & Wallander, 1988, p. 215)

This model reflects an underlying change in professional attitudes to chronically sick children and their families. Traditionally, research questions were framed in terms of identifying psychopathology, the assumption being that such children and their families were in some way deviant. Current views see individuals and families being faced with problem situations that they are unable to handle (see also Perrin & MacLean, 1988). These models also make specific implications about education and prevention. The task of professionals is to foster the acquisition of relevant coping skills, ultimately leading to greater independence and competence in dealing with stress. At the same time, the potential for psychosocial maladjustment and need for continuous professional involvement is reduced.

Population-based research

Several large-scale epidemiological surveys indicate that children with chronic disease are at a greater risk of maladjustment than healthy peers. Included in this approach is work based in Great Britain (Rutter, Graham & Yule, 1970; Rutter, Tizard & Whitmore, 1970), the United States (Pless & Roghmann, 1971) and most recently, Canada. In this latter work, Cadman, Boyle, Szatmari and Offord (1987) surveyed 1869 families in Ontario, Canada, including 3294 children aged between 4 and 16 years. The incidence of chronic disease was 14%, including 3.7% of children who also suffered from physical disability. (These data are broadly consistent with earlier epidemiological surveys, see Hobbs & Perrin, 1985.) Children with chronic disease and physical disability were at greater than three times risk for psychiatric disorder and 'considerable' risk of social maladjustment compared with healthy children. Those with chronic disease (but no physical disability) were less at risk: a two-fold increase in psychiatric disorder but little measurable increase in social maladjustment.

The epidemiological approach is clearly expensive and time-consuming. For this reason, most research is based on smaller populations of children, drawn from specialised treatment centres. The results of these studies are complex and suggest a whole range of outcomes, from no apparent effects of disease on adjustment to severe deficits. Many of these discrepancies can be traced to inadequate sampling, lack of or inadequate selections or control groups, or different testing procedures. A sample of relevant research is reviewed in the next section.

Asthma

Asthma is certainly the most common chronic disease of childhood in developed countries, and is associated with a significant amount of school absence (Hill, Standen & Tattersfield, 1989). However, absence rates are mediated more by social and economic factors than by the objective severity of the condition. Anderson, Bailey, Cooper, Palmer and West (1983) showed that variables such as poor maternal mental health, non-manual occupation, parental separation, more than three children and no access to a car were predictive of poorer school attendance rates.

Academic achievement in asthmatic children was traditionally argued to be superior to healthy children (Bakwin & Bakwin, 1948) but this has not been completely substantiated in later work (Graham, Rutter, Yule & Pless, 1967; Rawls, Rawls & Harrison, 1971).

Part of the difficulty in interpreting the results of empirical work can be attributed to the way in which the disease is clinically manifested. Renne and Creer (1985) have suggested that difficulties arise particularly because of three characteristics of asthma – the disease can be intermittent, variable and reversible in nature. First, asthma attacks vary in frequency from child to child, and for any patient, from time to time. A child may experience a bout of attacks over a short time, and then remain disease-free. There is much variability in the course of the disease. Some studies suggest that children 'outgrow' the condition. Increasingly, however, it appears that children who appear to have outgrown symptoms may re-experience them later (Siegel, Katz & Rachelefsky, 1983).

Second, asthma attacks vary in severity, from mild sensations of tightness in the chest or slight wheeze to 'status asthmatic'. The former is associated with slight discomfort; the latter can lead to death. Several attempts to classify asthma in terms of severity have been made, usually based on frequency of attack or dosage of medications. There remain a number of inconsistencies in the way in which objective severity is measured (Mrazek, 1986).

Third, asthma is reversible (McFadden, 1980). Children only experience respiratory disease during attacks; at other times their breathing appears normal. For some children, the symptoms of asthma are reversible when the children are removed from their homes (Peshkin, 1930; Creer, Harm & Marion, 1988).

Given these considerations it is hardly surprising that research concerned with whether or not children with asthma experience emotional or behavioural maladjustment, or even how adjustment levels relate to severity of the condition, has yielded conflicting findings. No relationship between adjustment and severity was reported, for example, either by Norrish, Tooley and Godfrey (1977) or by Steinhausen (1982).

In contrast, Mrazek, Anderson and Strunk (1985) compared 26 children with severe asthma aged between 3 and 6 years with controls, and reported that 35% of those with asthma showed emotional disturbance (compared with none of the controls). Those with asthma were also more likely to be depressed. Kashani, Koenig, Shepperd, Wilfley and Morris (1988) reported that 56 asthma patients (aged 7–16 years) did not differ from controls on a measure of self-concept, nor in the number or type of DSM-III symptoms. Parents of those with asthma were more likely to report that their children showed psychiatric symptoms (especially in terms of over-anxious or phobic behaviour) than were parents of controls. No relationship was found between the incidence of psychiatric symptoms and severity of the child's asthma (as assessed by medication).

These findings are broadly comparable with those of Perrin, MacLean and Perrin (1989). The level of psychological adjustment in children with asthma was similar to that of controls, and there was no simple relationship between adjustment and disease severity. Adjustment was significantly worse among those whose asthma was rated as 'moderately' severe by parents, compared with those rated as having 'mild' or 'severe' disease. While there is no conclusive evidence that children with asthma differ from controls in terms of adjustment, it seems that risk increases for those perceived by their parents to be severely affected, but it is not simply associated with more objective indices of severity.

Birth defects

Children with *birth defects* (cardiac disease, cleft lip or palate, and hearing impairment) showed behaviour problems two to three times the normal rate (Heller, Rafman, Zvagulis & Pless, 1985).

Cancer

The psychological adjustment of children with *cancer* continues to receive considerable attention. This is disproportionate in terms of the numbers of children affected by cancer compared with other diseases. However, significant improvements in prognosis as well as concerns about the potentially damaging effects of treatment ensure that children with cancer have a high profile in the research literature. Not surprisingly, given the seriousness of the condition and aggressiveness of treatment, children with cancer experience a highly disrupted school-life (Eiser, 1980; Spinetta & Spinetta, 1980). Psychological problems, for example in learning disabilities and academic failure (Taylor, Albo, Phebus, Sachs & Bierl, 1987; Mulhern, Ochs & Fairclough, 1987; Wheeler, Keiper, Janoun & Chessells, 1988), behaviour and adjustment (Wasserman, Thompson & Wilimas, 1987) and depression (Worchel, Nolan, Willson, Purcer, Copeland & Pfefferbaum, 1988), have all been reported (for a review, see Stehbens, 1988). A meta-analysis including 17 studies concerned with intellectual deficits by Cousens, Waters, Said and Stevens (1988) concluded that children undergoing CNS irradiation showed substantial deficits in IQ, and that this deficit was especially pronounced in those undergoing treatment at younger ages.

Largely because of the uncertainty surrounding the question of how radiation and chemotherapy might affect development, there have been efforts to assess psychological functioning of long-term survivors. While Malpas (1988) reported that achievements at school-leaving age (in terms of examination passes) compared very favourably with those of the general population, other work suggests that deficits are still present among children surviving more than 8 years from diagnosis. Peckham, Meadows, Bartel and Marrero (1988) studied 23 children who had been treated 8–10 years earlier. Children achieved less well than would be expected in reading and mathematics, as well as having difficulties in attention, concentration, memory, sequencing and comprehension. These difficulties appeared to be reduced for some who had received more extensive parental and school support.

Mulhern, Wasserman, Friedman and Fairclough (1989) also identified some subtle deficits. Long-term survivors showed a four-fold increase in school problems and somatic complaints of unknown origin over the general population. The presence of functional, but not cosmetic, impairment increased the risk of both academic and adjustment problems. Children who were older on diagnosis, were treated by cranial irradiation and lived in one-parent families were at most risk. Studies of survivors of childhood cancer point to the increased vulnerability of the group, and suggest that greater efforts should be made to provide appropriate education and intervention both during treatment and for considerable time after.

It is interesting that research concerned with children who have survived for short periods (1–2 years) suggests that those who are younger (less than 5 years) on diagnosis show more adverse deficits. In contrast, work with long-term survivors suggests that greater deficits are shown by children who are older on diagnosis. These findings need clarification. There are also unanswered questions as to the nature of the deficit in children treated for leumaemia by CNS irradiation. Some researchers consider the deficit to be global across all abilities, while others present considerable evidence of specific deficits in certain skills (usually attention, concentration, memory and mathematical reasoning). The nature of the deficit has considerable implication for the type of remedial intervention that may be most affected.

Finally, Greenberg, Kazak and Meadows (1989) have shown that long-term survivors of cancers and their families function within normal limits on tests of self-concept, depression, locus of control, family environment and parental distress, although scores tend to be slightly lower than normal samples. Those with severe medical side-effects (including cosmetic changes) had poorer self-concept, more depressive symptoms and a more external locus of control than those with no or moderate side-effects (obesity, short-stature, hearing loss, delayed sexual motivation or learning delay).

Diabetes

Diabetes is not traditionally associated with intellectual impairment (Anhsjo, Humble, Larsson, Settergren-Carlsson & Sterky, 1981; Kubany, Danowski & Moses, 1956). However, there is evidence that children who are younger on diagnosis are more likely to show intellectual deficits than those who are older on diagnosis (Ack, Miller & Weil, 1961; Anderson, Hagen, Barclay, Goldstein, Kandt & Bacon, 1984; Ryan, Vega & Drash, 1985; Rovet, Ehrlich & Hoppe, 1987). These deficits have been related to organic disturbance arising from multiple episodes of hypoglycemia. These attacks are both more frequent and difficult to control in young children (Golden, Russell, Ingersoll, Gray & Humner, 1985) and are known to produce abnormalities in brain function (Rovet, Ehrlich & Hoppe, 1987).

Adjustment problems have also been reported among children with diabetes, especially those in poorer health and from dysfunctional families (Johnson, 1988). It has often been argued that children in 'better' diabetic control show improved adjustment scores over those in 'poor' control.

Recent work challenges this view. Work by Fonagny, Moran, Lindsay, Kurtz and Brown (1987) and by Close, Davies, Price and Goodyer (1986) suggests that the efforts to maintain good control may be so demanding that children become more poorly adjusted (i.e. more depressed). Parents and doctors should be more aware of the highly demanding nature of treatment for diabetes, and recognise that many factors influence haemoglobin levels, rather than just the child's compliance (Johnson, 1988). There needs to be greater awareness that children with diabetes are unable to achieve normal levels of haemoglobin. Failure to acknowledge this can lead to unrealistic demands, and create undue anxiety and feelings of hopelessness and failure in children.

Haemophilia

Boys with haemophilia, like those with other chronic conditions, miss a great deal of schooling. Lineberger (1981), in a review of four studies, found that only 28–77% attended school regularly. Visits to hospitals, bleeding episodes and general illness symptoms account for these findings (Markova, MacDonald & Forbes, 1980). Studies by Markova, MacDonald & Forbes (1980) and Olch (1971) found that haemophiliacs tended also to have poorer achievement records than healthy classmates.

Notwithstanding the many tragic cases of HIV infection there have been recent improvements in treatment for boys with haemophilia. These enable more home-based care and should, in theory, lead to improved school attendance. In fact, amongst a group of boys receiving this treatment, school attendance was still relatively interrupted (Woolf, Rappaport, Reardon, Ciborowski, D'Angelo & Bessette, 1989). In addition, boys in this study showed significant under-achievement, especially in reading and maths. Despite improved medical care, and concerted efforts to integrate these boys into regular (rather than specialised) schools, much absenteeism and under-achievement still characterises their school-life.

Clinical observations suggest that children with haemophilia experience significant physical, emotional and social stress, all of which can be intensified during periods of exacerbation of the illness (Steinhausen, 1976). Wallander and Varni (1986) found that the average child with haemophilia showed more behavioural problems than 78% of children in a normal sample. Behaviour problems were likely to increase with age. In the same sample, Wallander and Varni (1986) found no association between adjustment and physical impairment. Disease severity (as measured by the percentage of normal activity of the clotting factor) was negatively related to adjustment.

Parents play a critical role in shaping the response of boys with haemophilia (Bruhn, Hampton & Chandler, 1971; Spencer, 1971). Haemophilia is an inherited condition, and parental feelings of guilt and responsibility need to be addressed. Madden, Terrizzi & Friedman (1982) reported a significant relationship between maternal distress on diagnosis and the child's subsequent adjustment. (For a further discussion of these issues see Chapter 5.)

Juvenile rheumatoid arthritis

Early work with children with rheumatoid arthritis resulted in very mixed results. Litt, Cuskey and Rosenberg (1982) reported that poorer self-concept was associated with a longer duration of the illness and a greater number of symptoms present at diagnosis. Ivey, Brewer and Giannini (1981) and Miller, Spitz, Simpson and Williams (1982) found no relationship between arthritis and adjustment. Finally, McAnarney, Pless, Satterwhite and Friedman (1974) found that children with more severe arthritis showed better adjustment (in terms of self-concept scores) than children with less severe forms of the disease.

A study by Ungerer, Horgan, Chaitow and Champion (1988) goes some way in clarifying these findings. Three hundred and sixty-three children and adolescents with arthritis were assessed to investigate the relationship between psychological functioning, social relationships, disease severity and adjustment. The relationship between these variables was dependent on the child's age. Adjustment in primary and high school children was related to psychological functioning and disease severity, but in the young adult group, adjustment was related to social relationships. For many adolescents and young adults, increased maladjustment appeared to be related to restricted social activities.

Some of these findings were confirmed in work by Billings, Moos, Miller & Gottlieb (1987) who investigated the psychological repercussions of both age and objective estimates of severity of arthritis. Objective severity was based on three indices (diagnostic type, disease activity and functional status). Forty-three children were categorised as 'severely' and 52 as 'mildly' affected. They were compared with 93 healthy children from demographically matched families. Psychosocial functioning was assessed using parent reports, physician evaluation and, if the children were old enough, self-reports.

Parents reported more psychological and physical problems for children with severe, compared with a milder, form of the disease. The severe group also had a higher incidence of school absence. As reported by Ungerer, Horgan, Chaitow & Champion (1988), older children participated in fewer social activities with their family or friends compared with control children, but this was limited to children with severe disease. Mothers of those with both the mild and severe forms of arthritis were more likely than mothers of healthy children to report that their children had difficulties getting along with school-mates. However, there were no differences between any of the children with arthritis and controls on measures of self-confidence or mood.

There is ample indication that difficulties arise for children with arthritis during early adolescence, and are associated with restrictions in physical and social activities. The implications for intervention would seem to be quite clear: increased social contact mediated by practical help with transport.

Renal disease

Among survivors of *end-stage renal disease*, maladjustment (as measured by distorted body image, social immaturity and poor self-esteem) was directly related to the presence of visible impairments (Beck, Nethercut, Crittenden & Hewins, 1986). Children with chronic renal failure showed significant psychiatric maladjustment (Garralda, Jameson, Reynolds & Postlethwaite, 1988) compared with healthy controls. Although more marked difficulties were reported among those with severe disease, those who were less severely ill showed particular difficulties in school adjustment and loneliness.

Sickle-cell anaemia

Adjustment problems, particularly in behaviour, social and personal relationships and body image, have all been reported among children with sickle-cell disease (Hurtig & White, 1986; Lemanek *et al.*, 1986; Morgan & Jackson, 1986). Difficulties have been noted to be more severe for adolescents compared with younger children, and especially for older boys (Hurtig & White, 1986). However, sickle-cell disease affects only black children, and failure to control adequately for cultural and social factors may have resulted in inflated estimates of the incidence and degree of maladjustment in these children (Lemanek *et al.*, 1986).

Like asthma, sickle-cell disease varies in severity. Again, as in asthma, there is no single measure of severity available. Physiological measures, such as proportion of irreversible sickled cells or platelet function, haematological parameters, as well as clinical markers (number of hospitalisations, number and type of crises or failure to thrive), can all be used as indicators of severity. Hurtig, Koepke and Park (1989) used a combination of measures as well as asking children to assess the intensity of pain experienced and frequency of painful attacks.

The results confirm earlier findings in suggesting that maladjustment is greater for adolescent boys compared with adolescent girls and younger groups. School performance was more affected for older compared with younger children. Global indices of severity did not predict adjustment. However, frequency of pain experiences was inversely related to school performance. Hurtig, Koepke and Park (1989) suggest that children who experience frequent pain should be monitored particularly carefully, in order to avert academic under-achievement.

Spina bifida

Spina bifida refers to a broad set of spinal cord complications. Different types of handicap are manifest depending on the specific lesion. Such variability needs to be borne in mind when considering the results of empirical research.

Laurence and Tew (1971) used teacher ratings of adjustment for 400 children aged between 5 and 11 years of age. Forty-five per cent were described as well-adjusted; 35% as unsettled and 20% as mal-adjusted. Much research suggests that children and adolescents with spina bifida are poorly adjusted (Dorner, 1976; McAndrew, 1979). They report feelings of loneliness, unhappiness and depression (Dorner, 1976) and have poor self-esteem (Hayden, Davenport & Campbell, 1979; Kazak & Clark, 1986). Wallander, Feldman and Varni (1989) found only weak or non-significant relationships between adjustment and various disease parameters (e.g. spinal cord lesion level, presence of shunt, number of surgeries, presence of external ulcers, independent ambulation and bladder control). Adjustment was, however, related to the number of surgeries experienced.

Studies involving more than one disease group

Very few studies have involved comparisons of adjustment between children with different diseases. Studies of this type are based on the assumption that maladjustment is related to specific demands of different conditions, which are perceived to be more critical than the general restrictions common to any chronic condition.

A longitudinal 5-year study by Breslau and Marshall (1985) suggests clear differences in adjustment between children with different conditions. Those with disorders involving the brain showed persistent and severe problems over the period, especially in the areas of mental retardation and social isolation. Children with cystic fibrosis showed improved adjustment over the period.

Other longitudinal work by Orr, Weller, Satterwhite and Pless (1984) was concerned with the stability of psychosocial effects of chronic disease over an 8-year period. One hundred and forty-four children with a range of chronic diseases were studied. Of 106 children studied on both occasions, psychological adjustment improved in 62, remained unchanged in 27 and worsened in 17. Children whose illness was associated with any kind of physical impairment showed significantly more psychosocial problems, centring round future plans, perceptions of family life and obtaining a driving licence. Those who had recovered from illness or showed no physical impairment did not differ from controls in overall adjustment.

Work by Stein and Jessop (1984) also suggests that psychological adjustment in chronically sick children is not simply related to disease-parameters. Both functional status (disability in terms of specific daily activities) and days absent from school were associated with poorer adjustment, but the association was relatively weak.

Wallander, Varni, Babani, Banis and Wilcox (1988) found few differences between children suffering from diabetes, spina bifida, haemophilia, chronic obesity and cerebral palsy. The children were reported by their mothers to show more behavioural and social competence problems than would be predicted from standardised norms (Achenbach & Edelbrook, 1983). Wallander et al. (1988) argue that the emotional demands of any chronic disease are more important predictors of adjustment than idiosyncratic demands of a particular disease. However, these data are based purely on parental reports of behaviour. Comparing the scores of children with chronic disease against standardised norms may be inadequate in terms of controlling for social class and other differences between the ill and general population.

Conclusions

Children with chronic disease are somewhat more likely than healthy children to show maladjustment, although the risk increases for those from underprivileged backgrounds (Anderson et al., 1983). The risk also appears to increase for those with disorders involving the CNS or physical disability. Parental perceptions of severity are more predictive of a child's adjustment than physician-rated severity or estimates based on drug use. There are indications that age affects adjustment. Younger children seem more affected in terms of school tasks and achievement (Allen & Zigler, 1986; Ryan, Vega & Drash, 1985; Rovet, Ehrlich & Hoppe, 1987), older children in terms of social adjustment (Ungerer, Horgan, Chaitow & Champion, 1988; Hurtig & White, 1986). Levels of adjustment also vary depending on the informant. Reports based on parent responses generally indicate more maladjustment than those based on teacher or physician reports, or indicated by objective measures (Kashani *et al.*, 1988). While maternal reports of child behaviour are a useful and valid source of information, they reflect as much about mother–child interaction as about the child's behaviour. For example, Lancaster, Prior and Adler (1989) showed that maternal health problems, marital adjustment and confidence in mother and wife roles influenced maternal ratings of pre-school behaviour. The association was especially marked for boys, who were more likely to be rated as aggressive or delinquent as mother's depression increased. Whether or not children develop behavioural problems is therefore intimately bound up with maternal expectations about normal behaviour and that of her own child. For this reason, maternal ratings of child adjustment should be seen to be as much a reflection of the mother–child relationship as an objective measure of behaviour in the child.

A second problem is that most empirical work has not taken account of the child's age in determining adjustment. Where the effects of age are investigated, it is clear that substantial differences in adjustment are found (see Ungerer, Horgan, Chaitow & Champion, 1988). Theoretically, it is very probable that age is a significant factor. This point is made convincingly by Perrin and Gerrity (1984). Drawing on the work of Piaget and Inhelder (1969) and Erikson (1964), they argue that physical illness has the potential to prevent or increase the difficulty of progression from one developmental stage to the next. The manner in which chronic illnesses modify developmental processes is dependent on disease parameters (such as severity, natural history, or prognosis) as well as social and personality characteristics of the child and family. At each stage of development, however, the child must master certain basic tasks, and ability to do so may be hampered by disease.

For example, during infancy, the main developmental task is related to the development of basic trust. Children with chronic disease may experience repeated separations from care-givers and painful treatments. These experiences may not be conducive to the attainment of a trusting relationship. During the period of 18 months to 2½ years or so, the basic developmental attainment is thought to relate to the acquisition of a sense of autonomy and self-control. Again, chronic disease is likely to interfere with the attainment of autonomy by restricting the child's control over procedures, medications or diet. Although this model is difficult to test empirically, the underlying assumption that we cannot consider adjustment without taking account of developmental change is very important.

Finally, part of the confusion in the literature lies with the inconsistent selection of outcome measures. However, in the absence of a generally accepted theoretical framework to enable predictions to be made about the kind of deficits experienced, this confusion is inevitable. More importantly, research needs to be directed at the implications of adjustment for the child or family, either in terms of disease-related behaviours (e.g. compliance with treatment) or for everyday coping and achievement.

5

Adjustment in the family

Introduction

Particular concern has always been expressed about the mothers of chronically sick children. It is generally assumed that mothers, more than fathers, bear the major burden of caring for the sick child (King, 1981; Tavormina, Boll, Dunn, Luscomb & Taylor, 1981). At least in traditional families, it is the mother who has greater contact with the hospital, who is responsible for ensuring that the child attends for check-up and out-patient clinics, and who invariably manages routine daily care. Mothers are often primarily responsible for giving the child daily medication, and certainly most affected by any treatment schedule that involves a change in the family's general way of life. For example, if the child needs a special diet, it is mothers who have to buy and prepare special foods, and perhaps make drastic changes in the diet of the whole family to accommodate that of the sick child. Otherwise, extra time is needed for food preparation, in order to provide the sick child with a diet which is different from the rest of the family (Acosta, Fiedler & Koch, 1968; Eiser, Patterson & Town, 1985). In some conditions, for example asthma, the child's attacks may be triggered by household dust. Again, this inevitably involves more thorough and regular cleaning, invariably by mothers. It seems that chronic childhood disease can create some very practical demands at a domestic level (Breslau, 1983).

At the same time, mothers have to juggle their responsibilities between the sick child and healthy siblings. This may be particularly acute at times when the child is hospitalised, and alternative arrangements need to be made for siblings. Mothers, more than fathers, may feel that the child's illness limits their opportunity to work outside the home. Few employers (at least in the UK) are sympathetic to parents needing time away from work to care for a sick

61

child. Breslau, Salkever and Staruch (1982) found that in middle-class families, the presence of a sick child reduced the probability of mothers working outside the home. This was not true in poorer or one-parent families, where the presence of a sick child did not reduce the chances of a mother taking on outside work.

The combination of additional practical demands and the potential isolation that can be experienced by women who are at home rather than in paid employment may take its toll on mothers' mental health. A considerable body of research suggests that mothers of children with the whole range of chronic diseases are especially prone to anxiety, depression and other manifestations of poor mental health. There is a general assumption that these responses are more typical of mothers than fathers. With few exceptions, it is not really known how chronic childhood disease affects paternal mental health – it simply has not been studied to the same extent. (In part, this reflects the unavailability of fathers at times convenient to researchers to collect data. Perhaps this in itself is indicative of the lower involvement of fathers in the routine care of the sick child.)

The literature that does exist points consistently to the fact that mothers of chronically sick children have poorer mental health than mothers of healthy children. Where comparisons are available, they also appear to have poorer mental health than fathers of sick children. This applies, for example, to mothers of children with diabetes (Borner & Steinhausen, 1977), cystic fibrosis (Gayton, Friedman, Tavormina & Tucker, 1977), spina bifida (Tew & Laurence, 1976), haemophilia (Meijer, 1980), physical handicap (Wallander, Varni, Babani, DeHeen, Wilcox & Banis, 1989) and epilepsy (Hoare, 1987).

Knowledge

Probably reflecting their lower involvement in day-to-day care of the sick child, fathers tend to be less knowledgeable about the condition than mothers. Johnson, Pollak, Silverstein, Rosenbloom, Spillar, McCallum and Harkavy (1982) assessed knowledge and practical skills (testing blood samples or giving injections) among children with diabetes and their mothers and fathers. Mothers were generally more knowledgeable than children or fathers (with some exceptions among adolescents with the disease). A similar pattern of response was reported among parents of children with cystic fibrosis (Nolan, Desmond, Herlich & Hardy, 1986). Again, mothers were better informed than fathers.

Mothers and fathers also differ in their perceptions of the severity of the disease, the extent to which it imposes restrictions on the child's life, and their understanding of the aetiology and prognosis. Mulhern, Crisco and Camitta (1981) reported that both mothers and fathers were more optimistic about the chances of survival for their child with leukaemia compared with physicians. However, fathers and children were considerably more optimistic than mothers. Levenson, Copeland, Morrow, Pfefferbaum and Silberberg (1983) also noted discrepancies between children and their parents in knowledge of cancer and perception of disease-related limitations. In particular, parents felt that children should be prepared to be more involved in their own care, and were concerned about the implications of behaviour for general health. For example, parents and children disagreed about the effects of tobacco, alcohol or illegal drugs in combination with anti-cancer medications.

Differences have also been reported between parents of children with diabetes. Banion, Miles and Carter (1983) found that mothers were especially likely to be concerned about the long-term consequences of diabetes and future complications.

Variables which determine maternal adjustment

Despite the many difficulties, both practical and emotional, which are encountered by parents of sick children, many appreciate the need to minimise the effects of the disease on all their children. Many parents learn to carry on life almost normally, allowing as little imposition of the disease on family activities as possible. As with children themselves, chronic illness imposes a risk of maladjustment on parents. The vast majority appear very resilient, and able to muster an array of coping resources and strategies to minimise potential distress and maladjustment. The emphasis in past research on describing the difficulties parents experience, and identifying the extent of maladjustment in the groups, has resulted in a paucity of research concerned with resilience factors. Yet the search to pinpoint resilience factors is not simply of academic interest. Understanding the processes and contexts whereby some parents come to terms with their child's illness and are able to provide a healthy environment for their family may give valuable insights for therapeutic practice.

The most systematic attempt to identify 'resistance' factors specifically in chronic disease has been made by Wallander and colleagues. Wallander, Pitt and Mellins (1990) outlined a model (shown in Table 5.1) to account for differential coping in mothers of sick children. Major *risk factors* relate to specific implications and limitations of the disease or disability, functional care demands and the associated psychosocial stress. The impact of these risk factors is thought to be mediated by a set of *resistance factors*. These include the socio-ecological, intrapersonal and coping factors (as outlined in the model of child coping in Chapter 4). Resistance factors can influence adjustment both directly and indirectly – i.e. resistance may directly modify the impact of disease by reducing the real demands of care. For example, mothers who feel in control and positively approach the challenge of raising a sick child may mobilise others, or equipment, to help them. Indirectly, they may perceive the situation as less threatening than mothers who lack these attributes. Similarly, disability or disease factors can also operate directly or indirectly. In the latter case, disease factors may increase the strain of daily care and psychosocial stress.

Stress itself can be moderated by coping strategies. Intrapersonal and social-ecological factors also operate in two ways. They can affect adjustment directly, or indirectly via their impact on the degree of psychosocial stress experienced and the quality and type of coping.

There has been no overall assessment of this model. Rather, it is argued (see Wallander, Varni, Babani, DeHeen, Wilcox & Banis, 1989) that the relatively small numbers of sick children treated in any one clinic precludes such an evaluation. Instead, a series of studies have been conducted to determine the impact of isolated, or small groups of, risk or resistance factors. In the review that follows, work by Wallander and others concerned with some of the key factors in this model is considered. Several factors have received little or no attention. Others have been investigated in the context of general family adjustment, rather than limited to maternal responses.

Risk factors

Disease and disability parameters

Disease parameters, such as severity, chronicity, or the extent to which the child's physical or intellectual functioning is impaired, might be expected to mediate maternal adjustment. Specifically, diseases that are more threatening or involve the mother in sub-

Table 5.1. *Conceptual model for research on handicapped children (Wallander, Pitt & Mellins, 1990)*

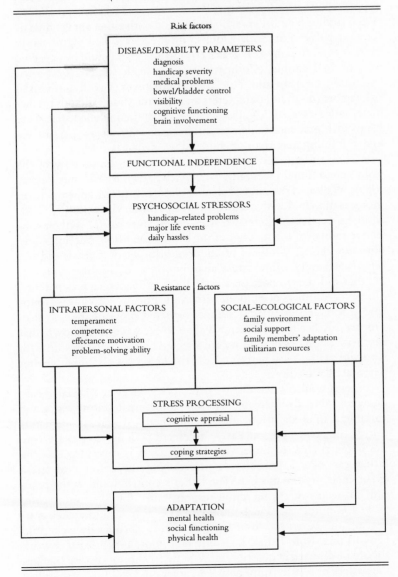

stantially increased amounts of care-giving might be expected to be associated with poorer adjustment. In an attempt to investigate this hypothesis, Wallander, Varni, Babani, Banis, DeHeen and Wilcox (1989) studied 50 mothers who had a child with either spina bifida or cerebral palsy. For both groups, mothers reported significantly more mental and physical health complaints than would be expected for a normal sample. (Comparisons were made with data reported by Rutter, Graham and Yule, 1970.) However, two hypothesised risk factors (disability parameters and chronic strain) did not predict maternal adjustment. Wallander *et al.* (1989) concluded that there seems little evidence to date to implicate specific disease parameters in determining maternal, or child, adjustment.

In contrast, mothers' subjective estimates of the severity of the child's condition do seem important (see Perrin, MacLean & Perrin, 1989). Walker, Ford and Donald (1986) compared adjustment in mothers of a child with cystic fibrosis and those with a healthy child. Mothers' reports of their own stress levels were related to their subjective ratings of the severity of the child's condition, but not to any objective rating. Mothers of children with cystic fibrosis did not report generally more stress than mothers of healthy children. Neither did they report greater feelings of inadequacy as parents. However, mothers of children with cystic fibrosis in two age-groups (pre-school and early adolescence) reported more depression than mothers of healthy children. Walker *et al.* have also shown that mothers' estimates of severity are affected by their relationship with the child's father, less perceived severity being associated with better parental relationships.

It seems unlikely that disease parameters, or even associated care demands, directly mediate maternal adjustment. However, these variables, in association with heightened care-taking demands during the pre-school and early adolescent periods, may exacerbate the potential risk to maternal adjustment. It is clear also that the father can play a crucial role in reducing the amount of stress experienced by the mother. The father's contribution can be practical, in terms of taking some responsibility for day-to-day care, as well as emotional. Much more work needs to be undertaken concerning the father's role in families with a chronically sick child (Tavormina, Boll, Dunn, Luscomb & Taylor, 1981). Related work should be directed at questioning if, or how, chronic disease changes the pattern of relationships between fathers and children, rather than neglecting the relationship altogether.

Resistance factors

Family environment

'Family resources' refer to a broad range of reserves and aids which are available to a family in time of need. These may be *psychological*, and relate to the way in which a family typically perceive and interact with both each other and the outside world. Resources may also be *practical*, and relate to income level and help that becomes available as a result of greater financial stability.

In terms of psychological resources, various factors have been implicated in determining either parental or child adjustment, or the relation between them, but there is little research of direct relevance.

In contrast, Wallander, Varni, Babani, Banis and Wilcox (1988) looked at the relationship between practical resources and adjustment in the families of 153 children, aged between 4 and 16 years of age. The children suffered from one of six conditions: juvenile diabetes, juvenile rheumatoid arthritis, chronic obesity, spina bifida, cerebral palsy or haemophilia. Practical resources were assessed in terms of income level and maternal education. These were compared with child adjustment and mothers' reports of family relationships (Moos & Moos, 1981).

Both practical and psychological family resources related to the child's adjustment. Together these variables accounted for approximately 17% of the variance in behavioural adjustment and 44% of the variance in social adjustment. Financial resources may be important predictors, especially of social adjustment, as higher income levels may enable children to participate in a greater number of activities outside the home. In addition, higher income levels are more likely to mean that families have the financial resources necessary for their children to participate in a variety of activities and cover the costs involved in travelling. Work by Anderson, Bailey, Cooper, Palmer & West (1983), concerned specifically with children with asthma, also suggests that adjustment is determined in part by financial resources, with higher levels of maladjustment occurring among children in families in poorer accommodation or where mothers have no access to a car.

It would, however, be dangerous to accept these findings without question, and see them as confirmation of the stereotype of the child with behavioural problems also coming from disadvantaged, or low-income families. Marteau, Bloch and Baum (1987) found no relationship between blood glucose control in children with diabetes and social class, family income, employment status or educational attainment of either parent. In fact, better control was related to psychological variables, such as family cohesion, emotional expressiveness, lack of conflict and mother's satisfaction with her marriage. It is clear that inadequate finances can add to the risk associated with chronic disease, but limited resources of this kind are not inevitably associated with maladjustment.

Social support

It was initially assumed that social support could directly ameliorate stress involved in chronic disease, with earlier work suggesting that families of handicapped children were often socially isolated (McAlister, Butler & Lei, 1973; Waisbren, 1980). Social support networks can be measured in a number of ways. *Structural* aspects refer to the size and density of social groups. There are indications that larger networks are associated with better adjustment (Hirsch, 1980). Families of children with spina bifida had smaller networks than families of healthy children (Kazak & Wilcox, 1984). *Density* refers to the extent to which members of the social network know each other, independently of the focal person (Mitchell & Trickett, 1980). Again, Kazak and Wilcox (1984) found that families of handicapped children had more dense networks than comparison families and that greater density was associated with increased stress.

In addition to these structural aspects of social networks, other more qualitative relationships can be involved. These may relate especially to the type of help that network members offer or the frequency of help given. In particular, the crucial variable may be the extent to which people *perceive* that help would be available should it be needed. Some of these qualitative distinctions have been identified, but not yet integrated in work with chronically sick children and their families.

An exception is work by Kazak, Reber and Carter (1988) who investigated social networks in children with phenylketonuria and their families. In addition to measurements of size and density, Kazak *et al.* also attempted to measure 'reciprocity' and 'dimensionality'. By this they mean the nature of the relationship between the focal person and network number (in terms of intimacy, friendship or acquaintance) and the kind of help that each person provides. Type of help was defined as emotional, informational, tangible (money, goods) or service (help with specific tasks).

There were no differences between families with a child with phenylketonuria and healthy controls in structural characteristics, nor in perceptions of the perceived helpfulness of networks. One of the few differences between the groups was in the extent to which parents included their spouse as a member of the social network. This was less likely in families with a child with phenylketonuria than in control families. This is contrary to the widely-held belief that families of chronically sick children adopt tight-knit or enmeshed relationships. Parents of children with phenylketonuria reported extended family members to be less helpful and to provide less emotional support than control families.

For all families, larger and less dense networks were associated with less reported stress, suggesting perhaps that this kind of network system is conducive to good adjustment in all families with children of pre-school age. Although social support may well mediate adjustment in families of chronically sick children, much more work needs to be done both in relation to families of healthy and sick children. Otherwise, we may be unable to assess the differential effects of social support networks in chronic disease.

Marital adjustment

Anxiety and uncertainty are inevitable consequences of childhood disease. There are increased practical demands of treatment in addition to the normal burden of child-rearing. As a result, parents often have less time to spend together. Further difficulties in finding a baby-sitter confident enough to care for a sick child often result in parents having very little opportunity to relax together away from the home. Many clinical observations suggest that the burden of caring for a sick child can have a strong and negative impact on the parents' marriage, resulting in a higher incidence of divorce (Lansky, Cairns, Hassanein, Wehr & Lowman, 1978; Tew, Payne & Laurence, 1974) and poorer marital adjustment (Crain, Sussman & Weil, 1966; Gath, 1977; Lansky et al., 1978; Tew, Payne & Laurence, 1974).

An excellent critique of this literature was made by Sabbeth and Leventhal (1984). First of all, they point to the serious methodological flaws in much of this work. (These criticisms largely parallel those that have been made earlier concerned with assessments of adjustment in children.) Control groups are missing or inadequate. Most studies are cross-sectional and therefore provide no information about changes in marital relationships throughout the course of the disease. Invariably, mothers are the only source of information. Little attention has been paid to paternal attitudes to marriage, to the child's disease or to child-rearing generally. Finally, outcome measures vary across studies, making comparisons almost impossible.

Sabbeth and Leventhal (1984) went on to review 34 studies looking at divorce rates and marital adjustment in families of chronically sick children. Seven studies involved children with spina bifida, six involved children with cystic fibrosis, four involved those with congenital heart disease, two involved those with cancer. Fifteen other studies were also included. Contrary to popular belief, the studies together did not indicate higher than normal levels of divorce.

Marital adjustment was found to be measured in a variety of ways. Some workers focussed on marital distress, others on closeness, communication, decision-making or role-flexibility. In contrast to the work focusing on divorce rates, discrepancies between parents of chronically sick and healthy children were found on all these variables.

While there is no evidence of a higher than average divorce rate in families with a sick child, it is apparent that there is considerable strain on the marital relationship. The factors which determine whether or not this strain leads to dysfunction or enhances and 'brings families close together' are far from understood.

General correlates of coping in families

Very little work has been focused directly on the identification of coping strategies used by children or their families in dealing with chronic disease. There has, however, been some emphasis on coping with leukaemia (see Koocher & O'Malley, 1981; Kupst & Schulman, 1988) and diabetes (Kovacs, Feinberg, Paulauskas, Finkelstein, Pollock & Crouse-Novak, 1985), with much less emphasis on coping with other chronic conditions.

A series of studies concerned with coping in families of children with leukaemia indicate a number of variables that are associated with 'good' coping. These include: openness in communication (Koocher & O'Malley, 1981; Spinetta & Spinetta, 1981), emotional support (Futterman & Hoffman, 1973; Kaplan, Grobstein & Smith, 1976; Morrow, Carpenter & Hoagland, 1984), quality of marital relationship (Kaplan, Smith, Grobstein & Fischman, 1973; Sourkes, 1977), family income (Koocher & O'Malley, 1981), religious beliefs (Chodoff, Friedman & Hamburg, 1964), 'positive' approach (Obetz, Swenson, McCarthy, Gilchrist & Burgert, 1980) and satisfaction with medical care (Koocher & O'Malley, 1981; Obetz *et al.*, 1980). Related variables were reported to predict 'good' coping amongst parents whose child had died. Spinetta, Swarner and Sheposh (1981) found that good coping was related to developing a philosophy of life, good support systems and good family communications. However, both Rando (1983) and Morrow, Carpenter and Hoagland (1984) did not find that social support networks were helpful.

Kupst, Schulman and colleagues (Kupst, Schulman, Honig, Maurer, Morgan & Fochtman, 1982; Kupst, Schulman, Maurer, Morgan, Honig & Fochtman, 1984) have conducted a number of studies to look at long-term coping with childhood cancer. In general, children and their families are reported to cope well, or even improve in the long-term. (Kupst and Schulman (1988) report findings from a 6-year follow-up.)

These studies point to an association between certain variables and adequate coping. However, the variables identified reflect the interests and intuitions of research workers, and are rarely defined from any coherent theoretical framework. The result is that some relevant variables have not been identified and no account is taken of the interactive effects of some variables. We are left with situations where, for example, social support sometimes predicts adjustment or coping (Spinetta, Swarner & Sheposh, 1981) and is not predictive in others (Rando, 1983).

This raises a second problem which relates to the definition of variables. 'Social support' tends to be used very vaguely in this kind of research, with no account taken of refinements in definitions. Social support can refer to the size or density of social networks, as well as individuals' perceptions of the amount or type of support available to them. Standardised scales are not always used, with the result that it is difficult to compare findings across studies.

A third problem concerns the definition of 'good' or adaptive coping. It is not a linear progression of growth without setbacks (Spinetta, 1981). Rather, families face a series of crises, and may experience many 'ups' and 'downs' in the course of coping with disease.

A number of assumptions are generally made by health professionals with regard to the natural processes involved in coping with any kind of loss. These assumptions are widespread, and apply equally to situations in which loss is incurred traumatically, by violence, or through illness. Individuals are expected to show an initial period of grief and distress, followed by a linear process of recovery. Some empirical work now challenges these views. Health care professionals tend to assume significantly more distress following crisis or loss compared with individuals themselves (Baluk & O'Neill, 1980; Wikler, Wasow & Hatfield, 1981). This overestimation of distress may be attributed to outsiders' need to preserve personal status and invulnerability (Wright, 1983). Society expects people to mourn in a predictable fashion. These expectations have been confirmed by empirical work, but little awareness has been shown for the wide variability in individual responses to loss.

Wortman and Silver (1987) present a considerable amount of other research which questions the assumption that individuals recover over time. There is evidence that some individuals continue to experience distress over extended time periods, and these distresses may be exacerbated by anniversaries or memories. Continued distress of this kind is relatively common and appears to be normal.

Work concerned with family responses to chronic childhood disease tends to be based rather narrowly on traditional 'stage' models of grieving (Bowlby, 1980; Horowitz & Kaltreider, 1980; Kubler-Ross, 1969). These models may lead to expectations that individuals must proceed systematically from one stage to the next, and failure to do so may be indicative of psychopathology. Other work in the area of chronic childhood disease is limited to defining correlates of 'good' or 'poor' coping. Our understanding of how families respond to chronic childhood disease and resulting ability to offer therapeutic help is limited by the narrow and traditional perspectives through which processes of grief and mourning have been understood.

Siblings

Children are inevitably affected when a brother or sister becomes seriously ill. Some may feel anxious that they are responsible for the onset of the disease, or even worry that they themselves will also develop the condition. Especially on diagnosis, siblings may feel neglected by parents and their psychological and emotional needs are often not met. Parents may focus so much attention on the sick child that they have little energy left for healthy siblings.

All siblings commonly complain about differential treatment from parents, and this is especially true for siblings of sick children. A common complaint is that parents are 'unfair' in their distribution of resources, time or sympathy between siblings (Crocker, 1981; McHale & Gamble, 1987). Siblings may resent special attention paid to the sick child.

At a practical level, there is a concern that healthy siblings may become involved in extra child-care or domestic chores (Powell & Ogle, 1985), although these seem to be modified by age and gender (Schwirian, 1976; McHale & Gamble, 1987). Lobato, Barbour, Hall & Miller (1987) found that sisters of handicapped children had greater responsibility for child-care and household tasks compared to brothers (although this difference did not reach significance). However, sisters of handicapped children received fewer privileges and were more socially restricted than normal controls. In contrast, brothers of handicapped children experienced more privileges and fewer restrictions on social freedom. The impact of chronic child-hood disease may therefore be reflected in changed expectations about the roles of brothers and sisters and associated family routines.

A central question in much traditional work in this area concerns the effects of chronic disease on adjustment in healthy siblings. There have also been attempts to determine disease or family variables that mediate sibling adjustment.

Some research suggests that siblings may become more compassionate, sensitive, understanding or mature, as a result of child-hood disease (Grossman, 1972). Ferrari (1984) reported that younger siblings of children with diabetes or pervasive developmental disorders were rated by teachers as more socially competent and positive than siblings of healthy children.

Other research suggests that there are no measurable differences between siblings of sick children and healthy controls.

However, still other work suggests that adverse psychological reactions, typically including aggression, poor peer relationships, low self-concept, anxiety, somatisation and depression, can be identified (Breslau, 1982; Breslau, Weitzman & Messenger, 1981; Ferrari, 1984; Lobato, Barbour, Hall & Miller, 1987; Tew & Laurence, 1973; Brody & Stoneman, 1983).

In reviewing this work, Drotar and Crawford (1985) conclude that (1) there is no one-to-one correlation between disease-type and sibling adjustment; (2) maladjustment is selective and varies with age, gender and outcome measure; and (3) in interaction with other variables, chronic disease in the family places healthy siblings at increased risk of maladjustment.

Lobato, Faust and Spirito (1988) argue that chronic childhood disease is a risk factor which may interact with other individual and family characteristics and resources to influence psychological development in healthy siblings. Their proposed model of sibling adjustment is based on the assumptions that (a) disease and disability characteristics and consequences are imposed upon and interact with features of family structure and function; (b) the interrelations of individual, family and community are critical to the study of sibling life; (c) many of the effects of disease or disability on siblings are indirect or secondary rather than primary, and, more generally, reflect interactional or 'systems' relationships (Lobato, Faust & Spirito, 1988, p. 403).

It is unfortunate that so much research has so far focused very narrowly on atypical sibling pairs and negative aspects of sibling relationships (aggression, hostility and teasing) while ignoring many altruistic and empathic behaviours. Siblings derive a great deal of mutual benefit from each other, and their relationship is an important precursor to peer and adult interpersonal functioning (Hartup, 1983; Lamb & Sutton-Smith, 1982). As Dunn (1987) points out, 'the sibling relationship is one of distinctive emotional power, passion and intimacy, of competitiveness, and of emotional understanding that can be used both to provoke and to support . . . It is a relationship of great significance and interest, one that contributes to the harmony or disharmony of the family and to the pattern of individual children's development within the family' (Dunn, 1987, p. 1). The significance of the relationship has only recently been acknowledged by developmental psychologists, and is yet to make substantial impact on method and theory in the context of chronic disease. Analysis of sibling relationships in terms of such concepts as aggression, hostility or maladjustment is hopelessly inadequate.

At the same time, it is necessary to consider the effects of chronic disease on healthy siblings in a wider family context (Dunn, 1988). Chronic illness may affect a healthy sibling directly (by limiting access to parental time or resources) and indirectly (by adding to general anxiety). There is some evidence that family characteristics and resources modify the psychological responses of healthy siblings. Ease and openness in family communications, the ability to adjust routines as necessary and work out problems together, have all been cited as critical factors (Daniels, Miller, Billings & Moos, 1986).

Family communication and interaction

Chronic childhood disease is a diagnosis that affects the whole family. In the final analysis, the responses of the child, parents and siblings are highly interdependent, and research which focuses on any group without taking account of the influences of other family members is bound to be incomplete. The focus of previous work on particular family members must be seen as a limitation stemming from methodological and statistical techniques, and not an adequate reflection of family life.

Observation studies by Minuchin and others (Minuchin, Baker, Rosman, Leibman, Milman & Todd, 1975) suggested that interactions in *some* families of chronically sick children differed from interactions in normal families in a pathological direction. More recently, Gustafson, Kjellman, Ludvigsson and Cederblad (1987) studied children with severe asthma and their families. Compared with healthy controls, families showed greater conflict, little ability to take decisions and rigid, enmeshed behaviours. However, this work tends to be based on clinic samples who are referred for specific problems, and therefore tells us little about the incidence or extent of problems in more representative samples of chronically sick children and their families. No measurable differences between normal families and those with a sick or handicapped child have been reported by Bolstad (1975), Tavormina, Boll, Dunn, Luscomb and Taylor (1981), Boll, Domino and Mattson (1978) or Spaulding and Morgan (1986). Undoubtedly, these issues are very complex (Garmezy, 1983). Many researchers argue that the only satisfactory method available is to observe directly family verbal and non-verbal interactions (Reiss, 1982).

Using this approach, Hauser, Jacobson, Wertlieb, Weiss-Perry, Follansbee, Wolfsdorf, Herskowitz, Houlihan and Rajapark (1986) compared 56 families with a child with recently diagnosed diabetes and 49 families with a child of similar age and gender who had had a recent, serious acute illness. In their procedure, child and parents independently responded to a set of 20 written dilemmas about parent–child issues (many were drawn from those described by Colby, Kohlberg, Candee, Gibbs, Hewer, Kauffman, Power and Speicher-Dubin, in press). The family was then brought together for a form of 'revealed-differences' procedure (Strodtbeck, 1951).

In this task, individual responses to the written dilemmas were revealed to the whole family. The experimenter then selected dilemmas in which three types of coalition had formed: mother and child against father; father and child against mother; or mother and father against the child. In each case, family members were then asked to defend their individual positions and attempt to reach a consensus acceptable to the whole family. Discussions were audiotaped and transcribed, and subsequently coded (Hauser, Weiss, Follansbee, Powers, Jacobson, Noam, & Rajapark, 1985).

The data suggest that differences exist between newly-diagnosed diabetic children and their families and control families (where the child has a limiting, acute illness). First, diabetic children and their mothers showed significantly more 'enabling' behaviours. This included both cognitive enabling (focusing, problem-solving) and affective enabling (acceptance and empathy). Second, diabetic children and their fathers expressed higher levels of constraining behaviour. This included both cognitive constraining (withholding and indifference) and affective constraining (excessive gratifying, devaluing). Hauser *et al.* (1986) argue that these results reflect important changes in family life following diagnosis of diabetes. Initially, families are likely to respond with a spirit of hope and optimism ('We'll fight this together'), and these attitudes of hope are reflected in increased enabling interactions. Other work by the same authors support this interpretation. Diabetic families reported higher levels of organisation and greater emphasis on recreational activities (Hauser, Jacobson, Wertlieb, Brink & Wentworth, 1985).

At the same time, families also experience more negative feelings of dismay, sadness, anger and guilt, which are less easily aired. This appears to be reflected much more in the interactions between fathers and children with diabetes than between mothers and their children.

Conclusions

This work may be of limited significance, with the findings applicable only to adolescents with diabetes. As yet, we do not know how interactions change throughout the course of the disease. The real merit of the work lies in an approach which identifies a range of interactive behaviours, some of which are supportive and constructive. Underlying these more positive approaches there can co-exist feelings of disappointment and guilt. The two are not independent, and serve to emphasise the complexity of human involvement and response to chronic disease.

Future work also needs to be directed at questions concerned with parenting the sick child. Specifically, we know very little about how parents modify discipline practices, or the demands and expectations that they make of their children. There is an assumption in much clinical literature that parents over-indulge and protect sick children, but there is no substantial empirical evidence for this. Yet parents must face a real dilemma in disciplining sick children; future work needs to investigate how parents make decisions and enforce discipline in families where there is a chronically sick child.

Finally, almost all the research is based on a traditional model of the family as a unit consisting of two adults and two children. Some estimates suggest, however, that 40% of children (born around 1970) will live in a one-parent family at some point before they reach 18 years of age (Bane, 1976). The difficulties that are faced by one-parent families are likely to be exacerbated by chronic disease. For example, Banion, Miles and Carter (1983) found that children with diabetes from one-parent families had most difficulties in maintaining adequate levels of blood-sugar control. Any completely satisfactory model of family adjustment in relation to chronic disease also needs to take into account the relationships and interactions that characterise one-parent families (Shapiro & Wallace, 1987).

6

Communication and education

Introduction

It has been shown in previous chapters that chronic disease can involve a major reorganisation in life-style for children and their families. Many families have little previous experience of hospitals, or the highly technological nature of modern treatment, and may well feel overwhelmed and inadequate. They are required to learn very rapidly about the nature of disease and procedures, and a whole new vocabulary that goes along with medical diagnoses. All this information has to be assimilated in as short a time as possible, while under extreme shock and distress.

Issues concerning communication and education therefore become of paramount importance. The manner in which diagnoses are made may well influence the family's attitudes to the disease, the hospital, and medical personnel, both in the short-term and well into the future. The family's response will also determine the way in which the child is handled, and the extent to which difficulties and maladjustments are anticipated or, preferably, a return to 'normal life' envisaged. The way in which a child is treated both by the hospital and by the family may be reasonably expected to influence attitudes to the disease and willingness to comply with advice and painful treatments.

Despite the central role assigned to effective communication, very little research has been directly concerned with issues of communication in chronically sick children. In this chapter, the advantages and disadvantages of open communication with child patients, and the way in which doctors do relate to young children will be considered. Secondly, research concerned with children's knowledge of their own illness is reviewed (very little is known about their related feelings). In general, this research suggests that children have very little information about their disease, and are often insufficiently informed to manage some of the practical aspects of self-care. In considering why this may be so, it is necessary to understand how children think about issues such as the cause and implications of illness, treatment and how the body works. Developmental changes about these issues are discussed. Finally, it is argued that such a developmental approach needs to be an integral component in any attempts at intervention.

The communication of 'bad news'

While there has been some research concerned with improving the way in which 'bad news' is given to parents (Greenberg, Jewett, Gluck, Champion, Leikin, Altieri & Lipnick, 1984; McDonald, Carson, Palmer & Slay, 1982) and documenting how parents react to diagnoses of chronic or potentially fatal disease in their child (Myers, 1983), very little is known about how such information is communicated to the child. Partly this can be attributed to the fact that such communications are restricted to parents in many cases, since it is clearly inappropriate to attempt much in the way of explanation to very young children. Partly also hospitals rarely have general policies on these matters, but leave decisions to individual consultants and families concerned. The result is that we know very little at a formal level about how explanations of chronic disease are given to children of different ages (Koocher, 1980; Spinetta, 1980). The dictum in many clinics is that 'children should be seen and not heard'. Doctors and parents may engage in lengthy discussions in the child's presence about the condition, but make little effort to include the patient at all. The result is that children can become quite anxious, and be given little opportunity to air their own concerns.

At a general level, we know that communication between doctors and paediatric patients is often inadequate. Pantell, Stewart, Dias, Wells and Ross (1982) video-taped interactions between a doctor, parent and child patient. While doctors made considerable efforts to elicit information from children, they directed almost all information about diagnosis and treatment to the parent. While doctors' efforts at communication improved with the child's age, doctors consistently addressed more remarks to boys than girls.

Two opposing views to communication with chronically sick children have developed (Share, 1972). This work has focused almost exclusively on the question of communication and explanations with paediatric oncology patients. The traditional or 'protective' approach which was favoured in the 1950s and 1960s advocated that children be shielded from full knowledge of their condition (Bluebond-Langner, 1978; Evans, 1968; Slavin, O'Malley, Koocher & Foster, 1982; Share, 1972). Such knowledge was assumed to be harmful in increasing children's anxieties and fears and subsequently interfering with effective coping (Plank, 1964).

Later research suggested that children were frequently aware of the seriousness of their condition, but also realised that parents and medical staff did not want them to discuss the matter openly. As a result, many children experienced loneliness and isolation (Binger, Ablin, Feuerstein, Kushner, Zoger & Mikkelsen, 1969; Spinetta, Rigler & Karon, 1973). The lack of openness also meant that some children fantasised about their condition, and consequently became more distressed than if they had been given the real diagnosis. Examples of this happening for conditions other than cancer have been given by Lindemann (1981), and Perrin and Gerrity (1981). Recognition of these factors led to a more 'open' approach, encouraging parents and physicians to share information about the disease (Novak, Plummer & Smith, 1979). However, very little is known about the kinds of information children are given about their illness, or the context in which it occurs. An exception is a study by Chesler, Paris and Barbarin (1986), who found that parents' decision to inform child oncology patients was based on a number of factors, including the child's age, sibling structure, religious beliefs and their own access to information.

Neither has much work been directed at the question of how knowledge of disease relates to subsequent behavioural and emotional adjustment. However, Slavin, O'Malley, Koocher and Foster (1982) suggested that adjustment to childhood cancer could be promoted by early and honest explanations. Children who were informed about their condition by the age of 6 years or within 1 year of diagnosis were better adjusted than those informed later, or those who learned about the disease by a process of self-deduction rather than direct information from parents or medical staff.

At a clinical level, it remains difficult to advocate that either a 'protective' or 'open' approach be adopted, until more is understood about how children interpret medical information and understand the relationship between this information and their own health. This is very much an area where developmental and clinical psychologists should work together, instead of basing practice on intuition or isolated clinical cases.

Children's understanding of chronic disease

Despite the fact that little is known formally about how doctors and parents explain chronic illness to children and that many patients are too young or too ill on diagnosis to understand very much about their illness, many researchers have been concerned to assess children's knowledge. This research is usually justified on the grounds that some knowledge is necessary in order that children can assume a degree of responsibility for controlling their own health. Children with asthma, for example, need to be aware of specific environmental or emotional factors that might trigger attacks, and those with diabetes need to understand restrictions on their diet and how to monitor glucose levels and inject insulin. In that diabetes demands a great deal of personal responsibility for self-care, much work has focused on assessing knowledge amongst children with diabetes.

Some of the earliest research was conducted by Etzwiler and his colleagues. Etzwiler and Sines (1962) asked 72 children attending diabetic camp to complete a questionnaire covering a range of self-care activities. Although 75% of the youngest group (6–7 years) could interpret the results of their urine tests successfully, difficulties relating this to their insulin needs were experienced even by the older children (16–17 years). Collier and Etzwiler (1971) reported that children most frequently made errors in relation to recognising symptoms of acidosis, testing for acetones, controlling their diet and understanding the effects of different types of insulin. Similarly, Garner and Thompson (1974) reported that a lack of knowledge of genetics, inability to calculate dietary intake and identify symptoms related to control were most common, especially for children in the 9–13 year age-range.

These early studies focused on paper and pencil assessments of children's knowledge, and tended to include a range of questions, some relevant to practical aspects of the disease and others more theoretical (e.g. 'Do you know what causes diabetes?'). Aside from the fact that there is rarely a simple answer to questions of causality, some of these more theoretical questions may have little relevance to how conscientiously children perform self-care activities. For this reason, subsequent research shifted in emphasis toward examining how well children actually performed self-care activities. Garner, Thompson and Partridge (1969) and Garner and Thompson (1974) found that children made gross errors in estimating appropriate-sized servings of food. Lorenz, Christensen & Pichert (1985) demonstrated that children could not select acceptable foods from a canteen menu. Malone, Hellrung, Malphus, Rosenbloom, Grgic and Weber (1976) reported that children lacked accuracy in interpreting urine results; only 41% of children's results corresponded with those made by laboratory technicians.

Similar inaccuracies were reported by Johnson, Pollak, Silverstein, Rosenbloom, Spillar, McCallum and Harkavy (1982). Errors in urine-testing were made by 80% of children; errors in self-injection by 40%. In both cases, children's skill in these practical tasks did not correlate with their scores on a more conventional assessment of diabetes knowledge. While older children were generally more knowledgeable than younger children, girls of all ages were more accurate with their practical skills than boys of a similar age.

In recent years there has been a trend away from urine-testing to self-monitoring of blood glucose. These methods are generally preferred by patients (Daneman, Siminerio, Transne, Betschart, Drash & Becker, 1985; Silverstein, Rosenbloom, Clarke, Spillar & Pendergast, 1983), and are thought to provide patients with greater flexibility in disease management (Baum, 1981). Patients are taught to assess their blood glucose levels by using visually read chemstrip reagent strips. Several studies have looked at children's accuracy in reading such strips (see Clarson, Daneman, Frank, Link, Perlman & Ehrlich, 1985; Wing, Lamparski, Zaslow, Betschart, Siminerio & Becker, 1985). Both of these studies report reasonable accuracy in children's readings. For example, Wing et al. (1985) found that 58% of readings were within 20% of laboratory values. However, accuracy did not relate to children's glycaemic control. Regardless of the method that children use to assess blood sugar levels, it is clear that they need constant monitoring and adult guidance in the interpretation of results.

Work with other groups of chronically sick children has also relied heavily on questionnaire assessment. Martin, Landau and Phelan (1982) reported that young people (aged 21 years) who had suffered from asthma since childhood were ill-informed about various aspects of their illness. They were especially badly informed about the potential dangers of over-use of broncho-dilators and did not understand the particular risks to asthmatics associated with smoking. Eiser, Town and Tripp (1988) found that school-aged children knew little about the aetiology of asthma, and were rarely either aware of or prepared to take actions necessary to avoid environmental or emotional triggers likely to precipitate attacks. (For example, children with asthma might report that attacks were precipitated by the family pet, yet take no action to remove the pet from the household.) Children and their mothers did not always agree about what were precipitating factors.

Other work with oncology patients also suggests that children and their parents may differ substantially in their understanding of the disease. Mulhern, Crisco and Camitta (1981) found that children were very much more optimistic about their prognosis than either their mothers or physicians. Levenson, Copeland, Morrow, Pfefferbaum and Silberberg (1983) studied 55 cancer patients aged between 11 and 20 years. Again, differences between patients and parents were noted on a number of issues. In particular, they tended to disagree over patients' self-help and treatments, the effects of alcohol, tobacco and drugs on the course of the illness and social issues concerned with how the disease was discussed with friends and relatives.

Inadequate knowledge of their disease has also been reported for children with cystic fibrosis. Nolan, Desmond, Herlich and Hardy (1986) found that patients were reasonably informed about treatment protocols, but confused about genetics and implications of the condition for reproductive risk and male sterility.

In summary, then, it is apparent that children with chronic disease can be poorly informed about many aspects of their condition. The finding that they lack information about the cause or physiology of the disease should not be surprising, and may have little implication for daily management or general health. Other findings suggesting that children do not understand practical aspects of their treatment are more serious, especially where this results in an inability to handle routine aspects of self-care (Johnson *et al.*, 1982). Among adolescents, there are particular difficulties associated with a lack of understanding of the implications for sexuality and reproduction on the one hand, and smoking, alcohol and drug-taking on the other.

Developmental changes in children's understanding of illness

There are several explanations about why children with chronic disease generally have insufficient information. They may be very young on diagnosis; people may, with the best of intentions, try to shield them from the resulting distress and anxiety; or the information that was given was available at the wrong time, or covered the wrong issues. As far as timing goes, it is unfortunate that the bulk of information is usually given on diagnosis, when children are least likely to be receptive and are often too ill to be able to learn effectively. Few hospitals are able to provide children with updates about their illness, or answer questions that may arise in the process of integrating treatments with everyday life.

Most research work has focused more directly on the question of the kind of information children would find most acceptable. This work is based on the assumption that children's beliefs about health and illness progress systematically through a series of stages parallel-ing the shift from pre-operational to formal-operational thought described by Piaget (1929), to account for development in physical concepts such as space, time or conservation. As a result, it has been suggested that children's concepts of illness are qualitatively dif-ferent from those of adults, and such differences need to be taken into account in communications with children. The argument has been applied to work concerned with (1) health education with school children (Natapoff, 1978; Michela & Contento, 1984); (2) expla-nations of acute illness and hospital admission (Eiser, 1984); and, in particular, (3) explanations of the cause of illness and rationale for treatment experienced by chronically sick children (Bibace & Walsh, 1981; Whitt, Dykstra & Taylor, 1979; Beales, Holt, Keen & Mellor, 1983). Implicit within the stage model are possibly unfounded assumptions and implications about the child's ability to understand illness and medical treatment (e.g. that children require a different type of explanation about illness and are *unable* to understand more 'advanced' explanations).

The cognitive stage approach to studying children's concepts of illness

Concepts of illness

Both Bibace and Walsh (1981) and Perrin and Gerrity (1981) attempted to describe children's concepts of illness in terms of a shift from pre- to formal-operational thought. Both developed question-naires, which focused on the child's understanding of the cause of several diseases, and beliefs about treatment and prevention. In both cases, it was reported that children's responses changed as a function of age. Between 4 and 7 years of age, children's beliefs about illness are dominated by thoughts of magic or punishment. Illness may be the result of witchcraft, or occur because of a failure to conform to adult instructions. During this period, there is also the emergence of understanding that illnesses can be contagious, though the child may over-extend this principle to assume that all illnesses are contagious. Children have little idea about the process whereby diseases are spread.

During middle childhood (7–11 years) children supposedly become more 'mature'. They accept a 'germ' theory of disease causation, and begin to realise that not all diseases are contagious. They acknowledge a limited number of causal factors in precipitating illness. At about 11 years of age, children realise that illness may be caused as a result of the failure of a specific body-part (e.g. diabetes occurs because the pancreas stops producing insulin). Around 14 years of age, some children recognise that disease can also result from psychological stress. Thus, heart disease may occur because the heart misfunctions, and because an individual overworks, or is subject to extreme stress.

Bibace and Walsh (1981) argue that children's beliefs about illness reflect the kind of logic that has been assumed to describe beliefs about other physical concepts, such as conservation. Thus, during the *pre-operational* phase, children attribute the cause of illness to magical reasoning or fantasy. From 7–11 years, approximately, beliefs are described as *concrete-operational*, because the child thinks in terms of mechanisms, but these are not stated at two levels of analysis. During the stage of *formal-operational* reasoning, from 11 years onwards, the child thinks in terms of mechanisms stated at two levels of analysis.

Concepts of the body

Gellert (1962) asked 96 children, aged between 4 and 16 years, to name all the 'things' inside them, to locate some of the main organs on an outline drawing of a human body, and to explain their function. There was an impressive increase with age in terms of the number of items named. Five-year-olds named about three items while 10-year-olds were able to list far more. The youngest children tended to think about the inside of the body in terms of what they could see or feel (bones and blood) or what they themselves had put there (food). It was not until 9 or 10 years that children regularly included items such as the stomach, lungs or kidneys. Reproductive organs were rarely named, even by the oldest subjects.

In parallel with the increase in number of body-parts mentioned was greater knowledge of the function of different parts of the body, and how these were interconnected. The 5-year-olds tended to assign a static function to each organ: the heart is for living, the lungs are for breathing, or the stomach for eating. Later, children described each organ in terms of its particular properties; for example, the heart is seen as a pump that causes blood to circulate.

By 9–10 years of age children build up a picture of the human body in terms of a system of organs involved in the movement of food, air and blood. Organs are seen as containers with channels of various sorts (blood vessels, food-pipes) connecting them. At around 11 years of age, children become aware that substances can be transformed within the body. For example, food is converted to energy and waste.

Crider (1981) discussed and extended the findings of Gellert (1962) and others (Schilder & Wechsler, 1935; Porter, 1974) and concluded that these descriptive changes in children's concepts of the body reflected a shift from pre-operational through concrete-operational, to formal-operational thought.

> Conceptions of the body interior begin with a global awareness of body functions and develop by increasing differentiation. There is first a differentiation of structure from function and of various functions from one another in terms of perceptual characteristics, then further differentiation of levels of body organization, specific organic substructures, and transformations.   (Crider, 1981, p. 56)

Concepts of death

One more example will be given. Pre-school children have been reported to regard death as a reversible process and deny personal mortality. Between 5–8 years, children become aware of the finality and cause of death, but only later do they acknowledge the universality of death. Stage-bound explanations of this type have been reported by a number of authors (Kastenbaum & Costa, 1977; Koocher, 1973; White, Elsom & Prawat, 1978). Koocher (1973) specifically related children's explanations of death to their stage of cognitive development, and suggested that concepts of death were dependent on more general reasoning processes. In particular, Koocher suggested that the acquisition of reciprocity skills (i.e. recognising the correspondence between individual and other's perceptions of the same event), which are supposedly developed during the concrete-operational stage, were central in facilitating children's awareness of death.

Concepts of related health and illness issues

It has been reported that similar stage-related changes occur in children's concepts of birth and sexuality (Bernstein & Cowan, 1981), medical treatment and personnel (Steward & Steward, 1981;

Brewster, 1982), health (Natapoff, 1978) and consequence of smoking (Meltzer, Bibace & Walsh, 1984). In practice, there have been few applications of this model to aid communication with children. Whitt, Dykstra and Taylor (1979), for example, suggest that explanations of illness should liken the illness experience to more familiar events. Thus, explanations of diabetes would suggest that the body is like a car in that both need fuel to work properly, and that the diabetic needs more frequent garage-stops than a child without diabetes. Similarly, an epileptic fit is likened to a wrong number or crossed wire in a telephone network. Work by Potter and Roberts (1984) and Eiser, Eiser and Hunt (1986) suggests very few advantages for children in being given such explanations over simplified medical information.

It has invariably been argued that research concerned with developmental changes in concepts of illness, bodies or death has practical application in explaining illness and treatment (Bibace & Walsh, 1981), and relates to the ability to cope with bereavement (Furman, 1970) and dying (Bluebond-Langner, 1978; Spinetta & Spinetta, 1981). An unresolved issue, however, concerns whether or not the course of development of these concepts in healthy children is predictive of the course of development in sick or dying children. In particular, it might be expected that the experience of illness, hospitalisation or death and separation might significantly alter developmental processes. While there is an assumption (see Bibace & Walsh, 1981) that experience will result in more sophisticated concepts, some empirical work suggests that fears and anxiety which may be associated with illness experience result in less mature reasoning (Myers-Vando, Steward, Folkins & Hynes, 1979).

Two studies have specifically investigated how children's experience of death or separation influences their reasoning about death. Reilly, Hasazi and Bond (1983) studied 60 children, aged between 5 and 10 years of age. A group of 20 had experienced the death of a close family member; a second group had experienced parental loss through divorce or separation; and a third group had no experience of death and came from intact families. Experience appeared to enhance children's understanding of death. Those who had experienced the death of a close relative gave more realistic information about death and the process of dying, but those in the separation group were indistinguishable from the no-experience group. The implication would appear to be that it is the experience of loss through death rather than separation which influences children's reasoning.

An additional finding from this study was that most of the children from 5 years of age had fairly realistic notions about death and acknowledged their own vulnerability. This may indicate that young, dying children are more aware of their condition than has traditionally been supposed (Debuskey, 1970; Ingalls & Salerno, 1971).

Certainly there are indications that, given a supportive environment and adults who are prepared and able to talk to children about their own death, young children have a great deal of insight (Easson, 1970; Waechter, 1971). Clunies-Ross and Lansdown (1988) studied 21 children between 4 and 9 years of age suffering from leukaemia. On the whole, understanding of death did not differ between those with leukaemia and healthy children. However, children with leukaemia showed a greater understanding that death involves the cessation of all bodily functions and is irreversible. The saddest finding was that the leukaemia children perceived themselves to be isolated in hospital – a finding that has been reported elsewhere (Spinetta, Rigler & Karon, 1973).

Criticisms of the 'stage' model

There is widespread dissatisfaction with the stage model as applied to children's concepts of illness. First, it is inappropriate for large numbers of children who do seem able to develop a mature understanding about their illness. Kendrick, Culling, Oakhill and Mott (1986), for example, showed that oncology patients as young as 2–3 years picked up a great deal of basic information quite soon after diagnosis. Although not formally informed by doctors, the children acquired information through observation and discussion with other children on the ward, and domestic and nursing staff. Second, the changes that occur in children's beliefs about illness may well reflect their personal experience as much as any structural change in ability to understand. It is quite common for parents to tell very young children to 'come in immediately or you will catch your death of cold' – a threat that may well generalise to a belief that illness is a form of punishment for wrong-doing. Later, when children first go to school, they are particularly exposed to a range of contagious diseases (chickenpox, whooping cough, mumps) and may therefore naturally infer that this is the mechanism by which disease is generally spread. Finally, children learn in biology lessons about the human body, and the role of risk behaviours, such as smoking, in the aetiology of lung cancer.

Developmental changes in concepts of illness may therefore be the result of experience and do not need to be explained in terms of a 'stage' theory. The fact that children of a particular age discuss illness in a particular way does not imply that they are absolutely unable to understand different kinds of explanations. It is possible to accept the descriptive framework outlined by workers such as Bibace and Walsh (1981) *without* assuming that the changes require any shifts in the kinds of cognitive operations involved. Related arguments are made by Carey (1985) who suggests that children's ideas about general biology shift from a perspective based on human behaviour (e.g. you eat because mum says food is ready, or you wash your hands before eating because everybody always does), to a more biologically based awareness (you eat to keep the body strong and well, or you wash your hands to prevent germs getting inside you). In addition, Carey (1985) makes the point that awareness of how the body works, or understanding of concepts such as 'animal' or 'living thing' should not be seen in isolation but reflect a much wider system of beliefs. By extension, we should not focus research on the relatively narrow issue of how children understand the cause of illness, but need to see development within the wider context both of real-life experience and growth in general biological knowledge.

In fact, the stage model has been subject to a great deal of research and criticism, none of which has made much impact on the way in which the model is applied to illness issues. Difficulties have arisen in explaining how the transition from one stage to another occurs, and indeed, regarding the very existence of such discrete stages of thought (Gelman & Baillargeon, 1983). The theory is generally criticised for the assumption that children develop within a 'vacuum', with little acknowledgement of the role of experience, and social or cultural factors (Nelson, 1986). Empirical work from a number of sources challenges the stage model (see Mandler, 1983), and even proponents of the approach have radically revised thinking about the nature of, and transitions between, stages (Levin, 1986).

Alternative theoretical approaches

A number of cognitive theories view the child as a 'theory-builder' (Rosch, 1978; Nelson, 1986; Carey, 1985). It is acknowledged that children have very much less practical experience than adults in all areas of functioning (Brown & De Loache, 1978), and that this difference in experience accounts for observed differences in the organisation and structure of information. There is evidence that adults and children structure information more similarly where experience is more related. Most extensive research has focused on how adults and children gain expertise at chess and in mathematical problem-solving tasks (Chi, Glaser & Rees, 1982).

The 'script' approach

In contrast to much work in the Piagetian tradition, Nelson (1986) argues that 'the key to understanding the child's mind, and thus cognitive development, is to be found by examining what children know' (p. 1). Nelson's basic premise is that representation of events is the fundamental form of the child's real-world knowledge. More abstract schemas are derived over time and with development. Thus, studying how the child organises everyday events may give insights into competencies overlooked in other research, as well as providing information about the development of more abstract cognitions.

'Scripts' are essentially schemata for episodes extended in time that contain representations of events that go to make up such an episode, and the *order* in which such events typically occur. Scripts thus generate expectations about what follows what in real time, and so help define what is normative or counternormative in terms of inter-actions between participants. From expectations of temporal sequences it is, comparatively speaking, a short step to hypotheses about *causal* processes. The organisation of scripts determines how events are perceived and remembered.

There is evidence that children as young as 3 years old build up sequentially correct, script-like representations of routine everyday events such as getting dressed, going to school or baking cakes (Nelson & Gruendel, 1986). These data very much challenge earlier views that young children are unable to order events sequentially (Nelson, 1986).

Empirical research on schemata and scripts has so far concentrated on issues of learning and memory, reading and comprehension, and (within social psychology) impressions of one's own and others' personality. The approach has not been extensively applied to questions of children's concepts of health and illness, with the exception of a study by Garvey and Berndt (1977). They investigated children's scripts of 'going to the doctor'. While children's knowledge of this event was less than their knowledge of other events studied (going to the store or on a trip), they did nevertheless show an ability to recall and order specific sequences as they might occur.

As part of a larger study to investigate the feasibility of using the script model to study children's knowledge of everyday medical events, we also asked two groups of children (20 5-year-olds and 20 8-year-olds) to describe 'what happens when you go to a doctor' (Eiser, Eiser & Lang, 1989). We identified eight discrete acts within the event (occurrence of symptoms, journey to the doctor, waiting, going into the surgery, being examined, diagnosis, journey home, recovery). Both groups gave well-ordered descriptions of the event, but the 8-year-olds included a larger number of specific acts. For example, a 5-year-old might describe the visit thus: 'We wait in the waiting-room and then the doctor looks in my throat', while an 8-year-old was more likely to include details of the journey and diagnosis: 'We get the bus, and then we wait outside till the nurse calls our name and the doctor looks in your throat and then he gives you medicine'. Thus, children of 5 years appear to have structured knowledge about the order in which events occur when visiting the doctor, and the order corresponds with that reported by older children. With age and experience, the scripts are elaborated, both in terms of the number of acts reported and the detail associated with each act.

The script approach seems especially suited to study children's beliefs about common-place medical events, and should be generalisable as an approach to study other related issues, such as going to the dentist, or hospital. It has an additional merit in being adaptable for use with younger children; it should be possible to develop a series of tasks to look at the emergence of medical scripts amongst very young children, using pictures and toys. Further work is needed to establish whether children develop a basic 'medical' script, which is elaborated to account for specific encounters, or if the various scripts develop independently. The problem of how different scripts relate to each other is, indeed, a fundamental problem in script theory (Nelson, 1986). Work is also needed to investigate the emergence of scripts as a function of illness experience, particularly in relation to how the experience of chronic illness and repeated hospitalisation is reflected in script organisation and structure.

Conclusions

Empirical work based on the stage model and concerned with the development of children's beliefs about illness has provided us with an adequate description of how healthy children think about a limited range of questions (cause of illnesses, treatments). Other issues which must be an integral part of the child's theory about illness (sick-role behaviour, preparedness to report symptoms or take medication) have been less systematically studied. The emphasis of the cognitive approach is at the expense of understanding social, cultural or interpersonal aspects of both attitudes and behaviours, in relation to illness. The descriptive framework may be useful in guiding clinicians in their initial attempts to communicate with children, but should not be seen as a reflection of children's potential ability to understand complex medical concepts.

Although a great deal of basic research is necessary before we really understand the processes whereby children integrate illness information derived from home, school, television and personal experience to form their own theories of illness, the work reviewed so far has made a significant contribution to our understanding that should not be completely rejected. It is clear that children attempt to make sense of illness experiences, and make inferences about the implications of illness if appropriate information is not provided. Doctors and parents should not discuss aspects of illness in the child's presence unless they are prepared to answer the child's resulting questions. There needs to be provision in all clinics for adults to talk together without children if necessary rather than talk in front of the child without acknowledgement.

Although some researchers have suggested that children of different ages require different kinds of information about their illness (see Harkavy, Johnson, Silverstein, Spillar, McCallum & Rosenbloom, 1983), it is doubtful whether such a stage-bound approach is generalisable for children of all ages, or even for other diseases. It is possible that the real limitation of these methods is in the assumption that critical information that children need relates to 'facts' about disease and treatment. In the next chapter, it is argued that this focus on facts is at the expense of other information that is at least equally important to children – how they view themselves and maintain self-confidence and esteem; how they explain their illness to others and integrate treatments with social and personal aspects of life-styles.

7

Intervention programmes

Introduction

Traditionally, interventions have focused on attempts to increase
knowledge and understanding of the disease and treatment. This
work is based on the assumption that increased understanding is
likely to lead to greater compliance with treatment, better
'emotional adjustment' and reduced behavioural difficulties (Blos,
1978; Dunbar & Stunkard, 1977; Rapoff & Christophersen, 1982). In
fact, researchers have generally been content to demonstrate
increased knowledge following intervention, and the implications
for emotional or behavioural adjustment have been left in the
balance.

Programmes to increase disease-related knowledge

Most studies have not investigated the effects of increased information alone, but instead combine educational techniques with
other behavioural interventions. Although there is some suggestion
that information alone can improve adherence to short-term medication treatments, it seems likely that additional factors are involved
in managing more complicated and chronic conditions (La Greca,
1988).

Nevertheless, increases in diabetes-related knowledge have been
reported amongst children attending diabetic camp (Shipp, 1963),
although more substantial increases occurred among older (8+)
compared with younger children (Harkavy, Johnson, Silverstein,
Spillar, McCallum & Rosenbloom, 1983). These results were considered to support the notion that children's beliefs about illness are
stage-dependent, younger children being unable to assimilate the
information as effectively as older children. As argued in Chapter 6,
however, such a stage-based interpretation is unnecessary.

Etzwiler and Robb (1972) used an automated teaching machine, and reported an increase in diabetes-related knowledge which was maintained at 3-month follow-up. Heston and Lazar (1980) evaluated a booklet for 7–12 year olds with diabetes. The booklet was associated with increases in diabetes-related knowledge, and again, older children (11–12 years) learned more than younger children (7–10 years).

Johnson (1988) criticised many diabetes intervention programmes on the grounds that a standardised approach is adopted, which assumes that all patients respond to the disease in a uniform way. For example, patients are often taught to associate certain classic signs or symptoms (such as tiredness, dizziness, dry mouth, etc.) with potentially dangerous changes in blood-sugar levels (hypo- and hyper-glycaemia). Recent work challenges the idea of such classic symptoms, and suggests instead that people experience these conditions very differently (Freund, Johnson, Rosenbloom, Alexander & Hansen, 1986; Pennebaker, Cox, Gonder-Frederick, Wunsch, Evans & Pohl, 1981). It is important to incorporate individual differences such as these into educational programmes.

A number of educational packages aimed at helping children manage and reduce the morbidity associated with asthma have also been developed (Creer & Leung, 1981; Scamagas & Rodabaugh, 1981; McNabb, Wilson-Pessano & Jacobs, 1986). Parcel, Nader and Tiernan (1980) reported decreased use of medical care services among asthmatic children who experienced a knowledge intervention programme. However, many programmes have not been evaluated at all, while others have been evaluated ineffectively. Rubin, Leventhal, Sadock, Letovsky, Schottland, Clemente and McCarthy (1986), for example, developed an asthma-specific computer game. While the game itself appears to have considerable merit and ingenuity, the authors compared its effectiveness against routine computer games. It is hardly surprising, therefore, that children who viewed the asthma games showed improved asthma-related knowledge.

As with diabetes and asthma, haemophilia involves a certain amount of patient self-care. In particular, patients are taught to prevent the potentially crippling effects of internal haemorrhaging by prompt treatment with factor replacement concentrate. Special care is needed to prevent loss of potency of the concentrate, infection, damage to the veins and spread of hepatitis within the family. Varni (1983) has suggested that patients' success with these techniques can be influenced by the kind of instructions given by medical staff.

Improved performance is associated with providing information in increments over time, organising the information in specific ways and combining verbal and written instructions. Although there is a substantial body of research showing that the success of any educational programme is dependent on variables such as these (see Ley, 1982), the findings have not generally been integrated in work with chronically sick children. There is also a focus on providing factual information about the disease. For example, children with diabetes may be taught about possible causes of the disease or incidence in the general population. These facts are not necessary in order for children to manage self-care activities effectively. For this reason, other intervention programmes have focused directly on teaching self-care skills and daily management.

Programmes to increase self-care skills

Self-care skills in children with chronic disease can be very poor. Johnson, Pollak, Silverstein, Rosenbloom, Spillar, McCallum and Harkavy (1982) reported that 80% of patients made errors in urine-testing and 40% in self-injection. Inadequate knowledge about self-care has also been reported for patients with asthma (Martin, Landau & Phelan, 1982; Eiser, Town & Tripp, 1988) and cystic fibrosis (Nolan, Desmond, Herlich & Hardy, 1986).

Again, efforts to improve self-care skills have focused heavily on management in diabetes. Various methods to improve accuracy in self-injection (see Gilbert, Johnson, Spillar, McCallum, Silverstein & Rosenbloom, 1982) have been reported.

Lewis, Rachelsefsky, Lewis, de la Suta and Kaplan (1984) compared two methods of teaching self-care skills to children with asthma (aged 8–12 years). A control group received 4½ hours of lecture presentations on asthma and its management. The 'experimental' group received five 1-hour sessions on the general theme of *active* control of the disease. Parents and children received separate interventions. Activities involving children were aimed at developing skills to increase personal mastery; parents were encouraged to create a home environment in which children could practice self-care and decision-making. Increases in asthma-related knowledge were reported for both groups, but those in the 'experimental' group also showed significant changes in self-reported compliance behaviours and a reduction in emergency treatments and days of hospitalisation. This study is exceptional in demonstrating that information in itself is of limited effectiveness. Children also need help to develop a sense of mastery toward the disease and confidence in self-care.

McNabb, Wilson-Pessano and Jacobs (1986) used a 'critical-incident technique' (Flanagan, 1954) to determine those behaviours which are important in the control of asthma, and can be managed by children between 9 and 13 years of age. Respondents (who included physicians, nurses, teachers, parents and children) were asked 'to think of a recent time in which a child did something that was especially effective or ineffective in dealing with some aspect of his or her asthma' (McNabb, Wilson-Pessano & Jacobs, 1986, p. 106). Additional questions were then used to probe for further information about what the child did and how effective the behaviour was. (A behaviour was defined as 'effective' if it led to a significant improvement in the child's asthma, and 'ineffective' if it hindered self-management or was detrimental to the child's health.) A total of 1374 descriptions of incidents were elicited from 565 respondents.

Four distinctive competency areas were described: prevention, intervention, compensatory behaviours and external controlling factors. Within these four areas, 21 specific categories and 66 sub-categories of behaviour were described. McNabb, Wilson-Pessano and Jacobs (1986) argue that these competencies need to be incorporated in programmes to improve self-care activities in children with asthma.

PREVENTION: These behaviours are necessary to avoid attacks or prevent the occurrence of symptoms. Children must learn to avoid precipitants, minimise the effects of unavoidable exposure and precipitants, take preventive medicines, keep medicines readily accessible, use some form of mental imagery to prevent attacks and cooperate with treatment.

INTERVENTION: These behaviours refer to actions that the child must take after symptoms begin. Children must take appropriate medication, leave the precipitating situation, practice any known intervention strategy, adopt this strategy according to the specific requirements of the situation and remain calm.

COMPENSATORY BEHAVIOURS: Children must adopt a variety of behaviours as a result of their disease. These may include dealing with peers, accepting responsibility for management, showing some determination to overcome limitations, cooperating with medical regimes, minimising the use of denial and self-blame, cooperating with painful aspects of treatment and avoiding manipulative behaviours.

EXTERNAL CONTROLLING: Adult behaviour was found to impinge, sometimes negatively, on the child's ability to manage asthmatic attacks. Authority figures may deny the condition, fail to provide appropriate help, interfere with treatment or use the condition to manipulate the child. Family problems may also precipitate attacks. In any self-care programme, children need guidance as to how to handle adults who interfere with effective self-management.

These data suggest that self-management in chronic disease is extremely complex, and programmes need to be far more comprehensive. A focus on adherence to medication is grossly inadequate. Instead, programmes need to address the wider range of physical, psychological and social competencies that are required, as well as dealing with the potentially negative influence of many significant adults.

Although increased factual knowledge about a disease does not seem to be associated with improved self-care or compliance with treatment (Shope, 1981; Varni, 1983), there is evidence that self-care skills are important. Parents' difficulties in handling therapeutic apparatus necessary in the control of asthma (Alexander, 1983) and haemophilia (Sergis-Deavenport & Varni, 1982; 1983) contributed to poor adherence amongst children.

The importance of both knowledge and skills in determining the quality of self-management and compliance may be age-dependent. La Greca (1982) found that parental knowledge of diabetes was significantly related to compliance for pre-adolescents, but not for adolescents. However, adolescent compliance was predicted from their knowledge levels. Other results also support these findings: children who are responsible for their own self-care are often less knowledgeable than children who are helped by parents to manage their disease (Eiser, Patterson & Town, 1985). It is clear that a number of factors other than the child's knowledge determine the degree of competence in self-care. Much more research work is necessary to identify the processes whereby children become self-sufficient in management tasks and to optimise the transition from adult-centred to child-centred care.

Certainly, there is no reason to assume that increasing a child's disease-related knowledge or self-care skills is necessarily desirable. Allen, Affleck, Tennen, McGrade and Ratzan (1984) reported that adolescents with diabetes who had a more sophisticated understanding of the disease and its limitations were also more worried than those with less knowledge. Intervention programmes which focus on increasing children's disease-related knowledge should also make provision to help them cope with the consequences of such knowledge.

Programmes to improve social skills

Adolescents particularly may neglect their medical care in order not to appear different from peers (Heisler & Friedman, 1981; Kagen, 1976; Korsch, Fine & Negrette, 1978). This can create difficulties for the adolescent with chronic disease (Greydanus & Hoffman, 1979; Simonds, 1979), especially where treatment is associated with cosmetic side-effects (Korsch, Fine & Negrette, 1978). Adolescent females, for example, may find it difficult to eat regularly in the presence of peers, since many adhere to self-imposed strict diets, in order to achieve a culturally desirable figure. It is difficult to suggest eating, if everyone else is desperately trying to refrain from thinking about food. In these cases, girls may be well aware of the dietary regime necessary to control their diabetes, and additional factual information would be of little help. Instead, helping the girls to cope with peer pressure may prove more helpful. This approach aims to teach children how to make others aware of particular needs associated with their treatment, without losing face or personal self-esteem.

'Social skills' approaches have been used in other contexts, including education about smoking (Botvin & Wills, 1985; Flay, 1985), illegal drugs (Eiser & Eiser, 1988) and sexual behaviour (Herz, Reis & Barbera-Stein, 1986). Social skills are primarily communicative in function (Swisher, 1976) and refer to the 'ability to cope with interpersonal relationships' (Argyris, 1968). A range of social skills appear to develop during adolescence, especially those involving assertiveness and the ability to agree and disagree, express opinions or make requests and initiate conversations (Pentz, 1980; Schinke, 1981). There are suggestions that individuals who fail to develop these social skills are more likely to show anti-social behaviours. Increased rates of delinquency, truancy, aggression and academic and social withdrawal have been associated with poorly developed social skills (Goldstein, Sherman, Gershaw, Sprafkin & Glick, 1978).

A variety of methods have been used to teach social skills. These include cognitive strategies for enhancing self-esteem, techniques for resisting persuasion, cognitive-behavioural techniques to cope with anxiety, verbal and non-verbal communication skills, and a range of other social skills (paying compliments, initiating social interactions, dealing with the opposite sex, etc.) (Botvin, 1983).

Several studies have used some of these techniques to encourage self-confidence and improved management of treatment among adolescents with diabetes (Gross, Johnson, Wildman & Mullett, 1981; Kaplan, Chadwick & Schimmel, 1985; Follansbee, La Greca & Citrin, 1983).

Gross, Johnson, Wildman & Mullett (1981) used a combination of modelling and role-playing procedures to teach social skills to four adolescents. They were subsequently reported to be more assertive in social situations, although the effects of the intervention on daily diabetes management were not assessed.

The other two studies involved comparisons of the social skills approach with alternative intervention programmes. Follansbee, La Greca & Citrin (1983) devised a programme involving six 1-hour sessions over a 2-week period, in which adolescents were taught to master diabetes-related assertiveness and problem-solving. Modelling, discussion and role-playing were used. These techniques were compared with an alternative procedure, which involved adolescents simply discussing disease-related problems and ways of handling them. Thirty-six adolescents took part altogether. Those in the social skills training group were subsequently reported to be more assertive in social situations. However, both groups showed improved treatment adherence.

Kaplan, Chadwick and Schimmel (1985) also compared social skills techniques against a method which focused on improving diabetes-related knowledge. The 'information' group met in small groups and discussed medical knowledge related to diabetes, learned facts through an interactive computer system and watched educational films. In addition, they made a series of video-tapes in which participants discussed diabetes with healthy peers. Four months after the programme, the groups were compared in terms of haemoglobin control and a variety of psychological measures. At follow-up, haemoglobin levels were significantly lower (indicating better control and perhaps improved compliance with treatment) in the social skills group. Other measures did not distinguish between the groups.

Perrin and MacLean (1987) used similar techniques, a combination of education and 'stress management', with a group of asthmatics. These children were subsequently less likely than controls to respond to stress with internalising symptomatology, and showed improved psychological and functional status (as reflected in time playing with age-mates and performance of household chores).

These four studies point to the feasibility of designing social skills programmes for adolescents with chronic disease. However, the studies were based on very small sample sizes, and more adequate interventions and evaluations are called for. In general, relatively short intervention programmes are reported. Interventions based on social skills methods used in other areas of health education tend to be much longer and more intensive. For example, Connell, Turner and Mason (1985) reported that 40–50 hours of social skills teaching were necessary to produce stable effects on attitudes and behaviour. (This contrasts with 6 hours reported by Follansbee, La Greca & Citrin, 1983.) A third problem relates to the implementation of social skills programmes: teachers differ widely in their attitudes and abilities to teach social skills effectively (Eiser & Eiser, 1988). Although this approach has tended to focus on adolescent health issues, it may also be applicable for work with younger children (Williams, Wetton & Moon, 1988). Social skills approaches to teaching children with chronic disease should also be extended to include younger children.

Interventions with families and schools

Programmes to improve participation in school-life

Children are generally encouraged to return to school as soon as possible after diagnosis of a chronic disease. Return to school can serve a normalising function on the family and signifies a renewal of everyday activities. However, physicians often under-estimate the difficulties that children can experience in reintegration with school-life after an extended absence. Children with leukaemia especially can experience stress in this context (Stehbens, Kisker & Wilson, 1983; Lansky, Cairns & Zwartjes, 1983; Eiser, 1980) and may subsequently develop school phobia (Lansky, Lowman, Vats & Gyulay, 1975). Difficulties may continue to be experienced long after the initial reintegration immediately after diagnosis.

All children with chronic disease are entitled to state schooling. However, parents sometimes have reservations about the suitability of this environment, especially for children who are perceived to be delicate or physically vulnerable (Turnbull & Winton, 1983). They also can be torn between the need to inform teachers about the child's disease and a wish that the child be treated as much like others as possible. Many parents fear that uninformed teachers will not make suitable allowances if the child feels ill and will be incompetent in an emergency.

At the same time, teachers have considerable reservations about chronically sick children joining their class (Eiser & Town, 1987). They rarely learn about childhood disease in regular training courses. They are very poorly informed about chronic disease and its treatment (Hill, Britton & Tattersfield, 1987; Bradbury & Smith, 1983), and tend to over-estimate the likelihood of medical emergencies arising in school. Teachers can also be uncertain about how to deal with the sick child. In particular, doubts arise over how far the child can be encouraged to take part fully in the curriculum, or how extensively allowances should be made.

Other difficulties arise in relation to healthy children in the class. Teachers are often concerned that healthy children can be made highly anxious and distressed by the presence of a sick child, especially where the disease is potentially fatal. These concerns, coupled with lack of information, can result in unnecessary restrictions being placed on the child's activities.

For many children then, it is necessary that attempts to facilitate re-entry to school are made. Crittenden and Gofman (1976) suggest that interventions should (a) help the child return to school, (b) deal with the social stresses associated with treatments and (c) educate teachers and other children about the disease and treatment.

A number of programmes have been described to help children with leukaemia return to school after treatment (Greene, 1975; Katz, Kellerman, Rigler, Williams & Siegel, 1977). Programmes directed at reducing social stress were described in the previous section.

Interventions with teachers have included workshops and seminars, and the distribution of leaflets. More imaginative techniques have been used with healthy school-children. These may involve formal lessons about disability, stories and films (van Westervelt & McKinney, 1980; van Westervelt, Brantley & Ware, 1983). Others have encouraged greater contact between healthy and disabled children over a period of time (Voeltz, 1982; McHale & Simeonsson, 1980; Rosenbaum, Armstrong & King, 1986), although few of these programmes have been systematically evaluated.

Armstrong, Rosenbaum and King (1987) paired gender-matched healthy and disabled school-children over a 3-month period. There was no formal teaching, but the children were encouraged to meet at least once a week. The children met at lunch-times and played informal games together. The healthy children were also responsible for helping the disabled child to come to school. At the end of the 3-month period, children's attitudes to the disabled were assessed and compared with those of healthy children who had not taken part in the programme. There was significantly greater improvement in attitudes among those who had met regularly with the disabled (as assessed in terms of willingness to interact). These effects were more pronounced for girls compared with boys. There were also second-ary effects on parents of healthy children, with greater improve-ments in attitude occurring for those whose child took part in the intervention programme.

While there have been a large number of interventions, aimed directly at the child with chronic disease, it is critically important to include the whole family in these efforts. The family is the child's most immediate source of socialisation, learning and support, and family influences in terms of coping resources, cohesion and adaptation, problem-solving skills and openness in communication are important mediators of child adjustment and compliance (Blotcky, Raczynski, Gurwich & Smith, 1985; Burr, 1985; Hauser, Jacobson, Wertlieb, Brink & Wentworth, 1985; Wertlieb, Hauser & Jacobson, 1986).

Family-centred preventive efforts should focus on helping the whole family to be involved in the care and management of the sick child. This entails flexibility in adapting treatment demands or ill-ness limitations within the established framework of family organis-ation and structure. In practice, interventions tend to be directed at sub-systems within the family. The parental sub-system is generally considered to be the most important determinant of child adjust-ment, and consequently receives considerable attention. Inter-ventions focusing on siblings or members of the extended family network are much rarer.

Interventions for parents

Interventions for parents tend to be aimed at facilitating understand-ing of emotional responses to the child's disease, and teaching methods of coping with practical demands of disease and treatment. Group therapy is popular as a means of contacting several sets of parents at the same time. The assumption is that a group setting may increase parental knowledge by exposing people to other view-points, enabling them to share emotional experiences and derive support from others in similar situations (Mattson & Agle, 1972;

Caldwell, Leveque & Lane, 1974). Detailed information about the organisation of parent groups was given by Saunders and Lamb (1977). Group leaders try to discuss issues such as aetiology, diagnosis and medical treatment, and offer help in the management of behaviour problems and psychological difficulties experienced by the child. Nimorwicz and Klein (1982) describe a programme for parents of children with haemophilia, covering basic knowledge, treatment costs, child-rearing difficulties, psychosocial problems and pain control.

Not all parents wish to be involved in support groups, however. Chesler (1984) reported that families were more likely to be involved when they lived within a short distance of the treatment centre, and when a child was diagnosed more than 1 year but less than 4 years previously. Within the first year following diagnosis, parents presumably derive some support from hospital staff. Perhaps also they feel unable to make new social contacts even among people with similar problems. Chesler also reported that women were more likely to be involved than men. This may reflect the findings, reported in Chapter 5, that mothers tend to take greater responsibility for child-care and treatment than fathers. Other research, reviewed in the next chapter, suggests that women are more likely than men to seek social support as a means of resolving stressful situations. Although support groups are highly acclaimed by some people, this method of dealing with personal crisis does not appeal to all. Greater provision of other kinds of intervention needs to be made for these people.

Interventions with bereaved families

The focus in most paediatric care and in intervention programmes is on living with chronic disease. While this focus is generally justified given the probable survival rates in most chronic disease, it is unfortunately true that some children do not survive into adulthood. Many young parents have no experience of death, and certainly never anticipated the prospect of their child dying. Therapists, too, tend to find special difficulty in handling their own emotions when dealing with the family of a dying child.

Spinetta (1982) suggests a number of issues that need to be covered when helping a dying child and family. Assurances are needed that the child will not be left alone; that life, while it was available, has been lived to the full; that crying, or feeling sad, is natural and acceptable; that death will not hurt; that there will be time to say good-bye;

and that parents will always remember the child with love and affection.

After the child's death, parents should be given the opportunity to visit the hospital and speak to medical staff involved in the child's care. Visits home by hospital staff should also be encouraged, to assure parents that they have not been forgotten.

Conclusions

Despite the urgent need to develop appropriate explanations of chronic disease and treatment for children and their families, many interventions are based on altruistic rather than theoretical principles. Others are taken from work with adult populations, with little acknowledgement of differences between adult and child populations in educational needs or abilities to handle information (Drotar, Crawford & Ganofsky, 1984). Many interventions remain reports of clinical case studies and are not evaluated beyond the specific situation in which they were developed.

It is also unfortunate that where interventions are evaluated, basic requirements of experimental design are often not followed. Inadequate programmes are used for comparison purposes, outcome measures are poorly defined and follow-up is usually of a short-term nature (Roberts & Peterson, 1984).

If interventions are to be improved, researchers need to define both the goals and outcome measures more precisely. Goals of preventive intervention may include: (1) mastery of illness-related anxieties; (2) understanding of and adherence to medical regimes; (3) integration of the illness and its treatment with everyday life of the family; and (4) integration of the child within home, hospital and school settings (Drotar, Crawford & Ganofsky, 1984). Adequate evaluation of any intervention, regardless of its aim, should not be restricted to global measures of psychological disturbance. Rather, specific measures which are relevant to disease management, compliance with treatment and coping need to be developed.

At the same time, age-appropriate programmes that take account both of children's beliefs about health and illness and their ability to handle medical information should be used. Interventions with chronically sick children need to be based more firmly within theoretical approaches which are truly developmental, and which take account of the potential contribution of mediating variables, such as family context and professional support.

8

Coping with chronic disease

Introduction

After the trauma of the original diagnosis, the problems faced by many children with chronic disease become rather less threatening. Stresses may be less dramatic, but tend to be continuous and repetitive. Practical restrictions imposed by the disease are one example. It is a nuisance for the child with diabetes to have to eat certain foods at prescribed times, to self-inject insulin or take drugs several times a day. It is a nuisance for the child with arthritis to find that simple tasks take longer to perform. Such daily hassles or inconveniences operate over and above those that all children experience. All children have to deal with school-related stresses (taking a test, being late, being teased, losing something important) and other interpersonal stresses (having an argument with a parent or teacher, being accused unjustly).

The purpose of this chapter is to consider developmental changes in children's appraisal of stressful situations, and the coping strategies available. The resources that children have available to cope with disease-related stress are necessarily based on those that they have found to be useful in other contexts. Our ability to understand coping with chronic disease and develop appropriate intervention strategies is likely to be enhanced by attending to normative changes which take place in children's abilities to cope with stresses generally.

Theoretical approaches to understanding coping during childhood

In the absence of a truly developmental model of coping during childhood and adolescence, most accounts have been based on models of adults' coping (see Lazarus & Folkman, 1984). At a very general level, coping refers to *all* responses to stressful events. Silver and Wortman (1980), for example, include in their definition of coping any instinctive or reflexive reactions to avoid threat as well as learned responses to aversive stimuli. For most purposes, however, this definition is far too general, and the emphasis in most empirical work is in defining coping in terms of *effortful* responses . . .

' . . . coping as constantly changing cognitive and behavioral efforts to manage specific external and/or internal demands that are appraised as taxing or exceeding the resources of the person' (Lazarus & Folkman, 1984, p. 141).

Lazarus (1966) argued that stress-management consists of three phases. *Primary appraisal* is the process of perceiving personal threat; *secondary appraisal* is the process whereby a potential response is organised; and *coping* refers to the process of carrying out this response.

Lazarus and Folkman (1984) further distinguished between problem-focused and emotion-focused coping. Problem-focused coping refers to problem-solving efforts or actions aimed at reducing stress; emotion-focused coping refers to efforts to manage the emotional aspects of the situation. For example, consider a child who has to attend a hospital for treatment. The child may attempt to cope with associated stress by demanding some control over the treatment, for example insisting that an injection is given to one part of the body rather than another (problem-focused coping). Alternatively, the child may respond by shouting, screaming and objecting to treatment (emotion-focused coping).

Although either type of coping can be elicited by any particular stressor, there is evidence that problem-focused coping predominates when people feel that something constructive can be done, while emotion-focused coping occurs when people feel that the stressor must simply be endured (Folkman & Lazarus, 1980). There is also evidence that the predominance of problem-focused or emotion-focused coping changes with age (Band & Weisz, 1988).

Subsequent work on coping in adults suggests that the distinction between problem-focused and emotion-focused coping is too simple (see Folkman, Lazarus, Dunkel-Schetter, DeLongis & Gruen, 1986). Carver, Scheier and Weintraub (1989) in fact describe 13 conceptually distinct scales which may describe coping:

Active coping is similar to the core ideas put forward by Lazarus and Folkman (1984) and described as problem-focused coping. It refers to the process of actively trying to remove or circumvent a stressor and ameliorate its effects.

Planning is clearly problem-focused, but involves thinking out action strategies and planning the necessary steps to handle a problem.

Suppression of competing activities involves putting aside other projects in order to handle the stressor.

Restraint coping involves not acting prematurely. Restraint coping may involve waiting for an appropriate moment, and from this point of view may be seen as a passive strategy.

Seeking social support for instrumental reasons is seeking advice, assistance or information, and is an aspect of problem-focused coping.

Seeking social support for emotional reasons refers to the process of eliciting moral support, sympathy or understanding, and is clearly an aspect of emotion-focused coping.

Focusing on and venting of emotion: this strategy may be functional, especially perhaps in mourning a death. Often, however, this strategy is seen to be maladaptive.

Behavioural disengagement refers to the process of reducing efforts to deal with a stressor, or giving up.

Mental disengagement refers to a similar process, and refers to a range of activities which can be used to distract the person from thinking about the stressor.

Positive reinterpretation and growth is a type of emotion-focused coping aimed at managing stressful emotions rather than dealing with the stressor itself. Construing a stressful situation in such positive terms should enable the person to resume active, problem-focused coping.

Denial is involved where a person refuses to believe that a stressor exists or acts as if a stressor is not real. As discussed in Chapter 4, denial can have a range of meanings. On the one hand, it can be seen to be useful in minimising stress and facilitating coping. On another hand, denial may make coping even more difficult.

Acceptance is especially important in situations where the stressor must be accommodated, rather than where changes can be realistically expected to be made.

Turning to religion: religion may be an adaptive response for some people under stress. People may turn to religion for several reasons: for emotional support; for help in positive reinterpretation and growth or as a means of active coping.

It is important to recognise that any single coping response may be adaptive for some people in some situations, but there are no universally-adaptive responses which are suitable for everyone all the time. Any response may become maladaptive if it is relied on for extensive periods or applied to a too extensive range of situations. Thus, it is too simplistic to assume that individuals adopt intrinsically 'adaptive' or 'maladaptive' responses. Rather, the extent to which a given response is adaptive or not is dependent on a number of factors, including characteristics of the situation or resources available to the individual.

In addition to this range of coping strategies, an individual has other *resources* available to cope with stress. These include related psychological resources, such as problem-solving skills, interpersonal skills and self-esteem. Individuals may also adopt particular *styles* of coping, which characterise preferred responses. These coping styles do not however implicate the presence of an underlying personality trait, but are consistent with personal values, beliefs and goals.

Carver, Scheier and Weintraub (1989) reported that individuals (undergraduates) were more likely to use active coping strategies in controllable compared with uncontrollable situations. In particular, planning, suppression of competing activities and seeking out instrumental social support were all more frequent responses in controllable situations. In relation to emotion-focused coping strategies, it was found that the more a situation was important to an individual, the more likely it was that strategies involving focusing on and venting of emotions, engaging in denial and seeking social support occurred. There was also a suggestion that people cope better when they are able to use familiar and comfortable strategies, i.e. those that are characteristic of their coping style. It is not clear what happens when individuals are in situations in which they are unable to adopt a preferred response.

Although developed to account for adult coping across a range of situations, this model could provide a very adequate framework against which to assess coping with chronic disease in childhood. It emphasises the complexity of coping strategies, and the total inadequacy of focusing simply on 'acceptance' or 'denial'. It also places emphasis on the process of coping, recognising that both the appraisal of a situation as stressful, and the resources available, can change with time.

Other coping strategies may also be essential to a complete model of coping with chronic disease. Information-seeking (Miller, 1987), assessing blame, engaging in social comparison or wishful thinking (McCrae & Costa, 1986) may also be used in these circumstances. These coping strategies need to be integrated with previous models of coping with chronic disease, while empirical work focuses more on the issues of potential adaptiveness of different strategies. There are advantages in adopting a general model of coping rather than developing models specific to the issue of coping with disease. In particular, this makes it clear that families coping with chronic disease are normal families, with an arsenal of available coping strategies which are applicable in a range of situations. Particular responses are not maladaptive in themselves, or even specific to coping with chronic disease. It is important to understand coping with chronic disease within a similar framework for coping with other stresses.

Some modifications need to be made in order to make the model applicable to coping in childhood. First, children are necessarily highly dependent on adults, and for this reason greater attention needs to be paid to the social context in which coping strategies develop (Leiderman, 1983). Adults can help or hinder the adoption of particular coping strategies by children. This was specifically demonstrated by McNabb, Wilson-Pessano & Jacobs (1986) (Chapter 7) in their study of children's coping strategies in dealing with asthma-related stress. Second, coping resources are likely to be tempered by psychological and biological preparedness to respond to stress. Differences in temperament may influence a child's responsivity to stress and the style of coping (Kagan, 1983), perhaps resulting in more responsive children having to cope with a greater number of threatening situations. There are also individual differences in how children respond to stress once they are aroused. Soissignan, Koch and Montagner (1988) report that on entry to school, some children show an increase in rhythmic stereotypies (rhythmic movements of parts of the body) and hyperactive behaviours associated with physiological indices of arousal. Third, developmental changes are likely to determine the kind of situations that children find stressful, as well as the coping resources available. Thus, children with chronic disease may find it increasingly difficult to handle the practical side of treatment regimens as they become more concerned with peer approval and their status in the peer group. With adolescence, children spend more time with peers and are more concerned with peer support (Hartup, 1989).

Work with children has not reached the same level of sophistication as that with adults, and still tends to be based on the distinction between problem-focused and emotion-focused coping. More subtle analyses as described by Carver, Scheier & Weintraub (1989) have not been integrated in work with children.

There are also reports of a relationship between different kinds of coping strategies and 'adjustment'. Compas, Malcarne and Fondacaro (1988) found that problem-focused strategies were associated with lower levels of maternal and self-reported emotional and behavioural problems. On the other hand, a preference for emotion-focused strategies was associated with maladjustment. Glyshaw, Cohen and Towbes (1988), and Wills (1986) both reported that coping strategies were related to adolescents' self-reports of depression, anxiety and substance use. There are also indications that children who cope less well with their disease are more likely to adopt emotion-focused rather than problem-focused approaches to dealing with illness-related stresses.

Spirito, Stark and Williams (1988) developed a check-list to assess 10 different cognitive and behavioural coping strategies. Two versions of this 'KIDCOPE' were made appropriate for younger (8–12 years) and older children (13–18 years). This scale was subsequently used to assess coping strategies employed by children with chronic disease (Spirito, Stark & Tye, 1989). The children were asked to think of a stressful situation which had arisen because of the disease, and rate the degree to which it provoked anxiety, anger or sadness. They were also asked how effective different coping strategies were perceived to be.

In dealing with disease-related stressful situations, girls were more likely to use emotion-focused coping than boys. In particular, they used strategies of wishful thinking and resignation and were inclined to seek social support. Boys were more likely to adopt a strategy of self-criticism. In addition, an increased number of hospital admissions and earlier age of disease-onset were associated with more frequent use of emotion-focused coping.

In a related study, Spirito, Stark, Williams, Stamoulis and Alexon (1988) compared coping strategies used by 47 children with chronic disease referred for emotional problems with 42 children who also suffered from chronic disease but appeared to cope adequately. Those who were referred with emotional problems reported a different pattern of coping strategies. They were more likely to use social withdrawal and wishful thinking than non-referred children. They were also more likely to use distraction as a means of coping with stress. (However, as a group, they experienced more painful medical procedures. The greater use of distraction may be a response to the stressful medical procedures themselves, rather than attributable to more general differences in coping strategies.)

There were also differences in children's perceptions of the usefulness of various strategies. Children who were coping well with their disease reported that cognitive restructuring, blaming and distraction were more useful strategies, while children in the referred group did not tend to report that these strategies were even potentially useful. Taken together, these results suggest that there are some differences between referred and non-referred children both in the strategies they adopt to deal with stressful situations, and in the appraisal of the potential usefulness of different strategies.

There is considerable scope for future work in this area. The findings of different coping strategies used by referred and non-referred children need replication. It is also necessary to explore the value of coping strategies in relation to specific disease-related stresses, i.e. are some strategies more useful in dealing with associated interpersonal stresses? To what extent are strategies determined by characteristics of a disease or its limitations? Diseases that are unpredictable, or respond poorly to treatment, may be particularly conducive to the development of emotion-focused coping responses. Research also needs to be directed at the question of how effectively children are able to rely on strategies developed in other contexts to deal with disease-related situations.

By implication, interventions should help children appraise the potential stress associated with any situation, and help them understand the different ways in which it may be handled. They need to accept that it is sometimes possible to fall back on preferred ways of coping, rather than acquire new skills, but no single coping strategy (or small group of strategies) is appropriate across a range of situations. A coping approach should emphasise the continuities between coping with disease and other everyday stresses, rather than emphasise the disparities.

Coping with everyday stress

Aside from this work by Spirito and his colleagues on children coping with chronic disease, and work reviewed in Chapter 3 concerned with coping with painful treatments, little is known about how they manage more everyday stresses associated with their disease. The remainder of this chapter is concerned with this issue, and with how understanding developmental changes in coping processes generally may help us describe and explain coping with illness-related problems.

Interpersonal stress

Chronic disease is likely to impose considerable demands on the child's interpersonal problem-solving skills. It may be necessary to justify school absence, apparent favouritism by teachers or being allowed to eat snacks during the course of a lesson. All of these situations may create resentments on the part of other children. Certainly there are indications in the literature that chronically sick children can appear socially isolated. Reports concerning oncology patients especially suggest that many are subject to unnecessary and unacceptable levels of teasing (Ross & Ross, 1984b). Helping children develop interpersonal skills which enable them to handle these situations is very necessary. There is some evidence that teaching children interpersonal skills leads to improvements in behaviour amongst previously maladjusted children (Spivack & Shure, 1982). As discussed in Chapter 7, it has also been reported that this kind of teaching is successful in helping diabetic children handle interpersonal stress (Gross, Johnson, Wildman & Mullett, 1981).

The most significant work in this area has been conducted by Spivack, Shure and their colleagues (Spivack & Shure, 1985). Their concern has been with how children and adolescents recognise and think during interpersonal encounters. A range of interpersonal cognitive problem-solving skills have been identified (generation of alternative solutions; consideration of the consequences of social acts; development of means–ends thinking; development of social-causal reasoning; sensitivity to problems and a dynamic orientation; Spivack & Shure, 1985).

Empirical work has demonstrated that these skills emerge at different points in development. By 4–5 years of age, children develop the ability to generate alternative solutions to many problems, and this remains an essential component of interpersonal problem-solving skills throughout life. Other skills emerge much later. For example, the development of means–ends thinking (mentally identifying the sequence of acts necessary to achieve a particular solution) does not appear until 8–10 years. Thus, at least in an interpersonal context, the skills available to children to cope with stress differ significantly as a function of age. Spivack and Shure (1982) have further reported a relationship between available coping skills and an individual's social adjustment. Again, interventions with chronically sick children need to take into account differences in coping resources.

School-related stress

The literature on coping with stress and failure in school is especially relevant when dealing with chronically sick children. There seems little doubt that these children experience higher than average absenteeism. For example, Fowler, Johnson and Atkinson (1985) studied school absence and achievement in 270 children with chronic health conditions. The mean number of days school missed was 16, compared with less than 7 days for the rest of the school population (in North Carolina). School achievement was predicted by the number of clinic visits, physician ratings of restrictions on activity, gender (girls were absent more than boys) and specific health conditions. Those with spina bifida, sickle-cell disease or epilepsy, and those from lower socioeconomic families, had particularly low achievement scores, although none of these variables predicted school absence. Other authors, too, have noted reduced academic attainments (see Mearig, 1985; Eiser, 1986).

It is almost inevitable that young children experience interrupted schooling following diagnosis, and their academic attainments suffer. The importance of these findings is not only relevant to the child's current academic achievements, but also has implications for how children manage stress throughout their school life. Work by Dweck and colleagues suggests that for some children, at least, early school failure results in a cycle of despair and poor achievement.

The work of Dweck and colleagues parallels that of Spivack and Shure, but is concentrated on identifying children's responses to stressful situations in school. Dweck and Wortman (1982) argue that children differ substantially in their responses to school failure. On the one hand, 'mastery-orientated' children appear to be effective copers. In general, they sustain high levels of motivation, persist at attempts at problem-solving, increase their concentration and display enhanced performances. On the other hand, 'helpless' children appear to be inefficient copers. This is reflected in reduced levels of effort, high levels of discouragement and deteriorating performance. Prior to failure the two groups do not appear to be distinguishable, but the cognitive coping strategies employed in response to failure differ markedly (Dweck & Licht, 1980). Mastery-orientated children attribute success to their own abilities and failure to changeable factors such as effort, while helpless children blame their failure on a lack of personal ability and see success in relation to variable factors (Dweck & Reppucci, 1973). The attribution pattern of helpless children was found to occur more often in girls than boys and has been linked to socialisation processes in the classroom (Dweck, Guetz & Strauss, 1980).

In subsequent work, it has been suggested that the key difference between mastery-orientated and helpless children is less in the types of attributions they make regarding failure, and more with whether they generate any attributions at all. Mastery-orientated children were less likely to generate self-attributions about failure, but instead focused on developing problem-solving strategies, and generating alternative solutions and task-related information. Helpless children tended to focus on the reasons for the failure, and were especially likely to do this in a self-derogatory way.

It is important to recognise that chronic disease may increase the probability that a child will experience school failure, both academically and at an interpersonal level. There are, however, difficulties in seeing this failure purely, or predominantly, in relation to a child's disease. In this case, attempts at intervention focus on making available some kind of remedial teaching, and helping the child reach similar attainment levels as the rest of the class. Academic failure, however, may have greater implications, in terms of distorting the child's attitude to school-work and perceptions of goals.

It is therefore necessary to see school failure, whether or not it can be attributed to chronic disease, in terms of a wider and more general theoretical framework, as, for example, outlined by Dweck and colleagues. This makes it clear that the child's difficulties are shared by others, and cannot be attributable to some pathological disease process. There are also implications about intervention. It is necessary to direct such efforts not only toward boosting academic achievement, but also toward helping the child redefine the purpose and goals of education. Such an approach is more likely to have long-term implications in shaping the child's attitudes to coping in any achievement-related situation, rather than be limited within the school setting.

Conclusions

There is evidence that interpersonal and achievement-orientated coping strategies develop throughout childhood, and are influenced by environmental and personality factors. How a child copes with chronic disease is determined in part by the child's age, gender and acquired coping skills. It is essential to see coping with chronic disease within a similar framework to that developed to account for coping in more general contexts. This ensures that interventions are age-appropriate. For example, Spivack and Shure (1985) have shown that the mental ability to identify a sequence of acts necessary to reach a particular goal does not develop until 8–10 years of age. These kinds of restrictions in reasoning should be kept in mind in devising interventions.

'Coping' is a broadly defined term, which is not used consistently in the literature on childhood disease. It is often inferred from parents' responses to individual items on general questionnaires, and as such it is often not possible to make comparisons across different studies. Recent standardised questionnaires that assess child (Spirito, Stark & Williams, 1988) and adult (see Carver, Scheier & Weintraub, 1989) coping should be adopted more routinely.

9

Future directions

Developmental perspectives

One of the central themes in this book has been that issues of coping and adjustment to chronic childhood disease should be understood within a developmental framework. In fact, many theories and methods have been based on work with adults, and extrapolated to child populations. Research concerned with child health and illness behaviour can be embedded in assumptions about the implications of child health behaviours and attitudes for adult functioning, rather than seen to be of interest in their own right. For example, the goal of much anti-smoking propaganda may be to reduce the incidence of chronic disease and mortality in adults; the goal of diabetes-education programmes is often defined in terms of reducing the probability of long-term complications (such as blindness or vascular problems). In both cases, the rationale behind the education programmes is in terms of the effects on adult health; any repercussions for child health are considered incidental. This orientation seems to regard issues of child health as an after-thought, almost secondary to the key concern about adult health. Interventions may be developed primarily for adult groups, and later translated as well as possible for practice with children.

This approach is, of course, highly defensible in many ways. However, it is not the only way to proceed, and the focus on adult issues may lead to insufficient attention being paid to specific childhood concerns. The alternative is to begin from a developmental perspective.

> One might also begin with theory and research in the nature of specific childhood problems and then consider the extent to which developmental changes and domains of functioning (e.g. affect and

cognition) may influence the emergence or amelioration of the dysfunction. On the basis of these sources of information, specific
techniques might be developed for children.   (Kazdin, 1989, p. 186)

This view had been elaborated by others, most notably by
Maddux and colleagues. Maddux, Roberts, Sleddon and Wright
(1986) argued that developments in motor, cognitive and psychosocial skills are related to:

(1) exposure to health hazards;
(2) understanding the causal relationships between behaviour and
     health or illness;
(3) ability to act on one's own behalf and assume responsibility for
     health and safety;
(4) behavioural and emotional responses to illness and injury;
(5) types of intervention and prevention strategies that are most
     effective; and
(6) times at which these strategies are most likely to be effective.

Thus, there are changes in the type of accidents experienced by
children and which appear to be influenced by motor development
and associated increases in mobility. Children between 1 and 4 years
have higher rates of accidental poisoning; those between 5 and 9
years have higher rates of pedestrian accidents and older children and
adolescents have the highest rates of accidents involving recreational
equipment (see Califano, 1979). There are developmental changes,
too, in common illness experiences. Particularly during the primary
school period, the most common illnesses to affect children are the
contagious acute infections, such as chickenpox and German
measles. There are developmental changes in children's preparedness to report symptoms (Lewis & Lewis, 1982) and understanding
of the causes, treatment and implications of illness. There are
changes, too, in compliance with health regimes (Varni & Jay, 1984),
and attitudes towards pain (McGrath & Unruh, 1987).

At the same time, there are developmental changes in the kinds of
health education programmes that are most appropriate, both in
terms of content and activity level. Active participation (e.g. role
playing or guided practice) enhances performance for younger children, at least in programmes to improve tooth-brushing techniques
(Claerhout & Lutzker, 1981) and safety behaviour (Jones, Kazdin &
Haney, 1981). There are also suggestions that the kinds of information about disease that are most appropriate are also age-related
(Harkavy et al., 1983).

Structuralist versus functionalist approaches

The danger in adopting a developmental approach is that it is invariably assumed to be a 'stage' approach. Thus, it is argued that cognitive understanding of health, illness and related issues is stage-related (Bibace & Walsh, 1981). Emotional consequences of chronic disease, also, have been described in terms of a stage model (Perrin & Gerity, 1984; Karoly, 1982). However adequate these results may be at a descriptive level, explanations are not dependent on the existence of cognitive operations.

There are several difficulties with the stage model. First, there has been much theoretical criticism. The model takes no account of social or cultural influences on development; neither does it account for transitions between stages (Gelman & Baillargeon, 1983; Mandler, 1983). Second, much empirical data does not fit theoretical predictions. There is little evidence of the existence of discrete stages. Mandler (1983) has argued that there is no quantifiable transition between pre-operational and concrete-operational stages. In addition, children can show responses characteristic of more than one stage at the same time. Altering instructions or details of the task demands substantially influences children's responses. Many research paradigms involve extensive and repetitive questioning which is divorced from everyday discourse; children may well feel confused and misinterpret the purpose of the interviewer's questions. Third, even proponents of the stage model recognise that some refinements need to be made to account for theoretical criticisms and empirical data (Levin, 1986). These refinements have not been included in any 'stage' accounts of illness beliefs or understanding. Rather, researchers have relied on rather simplified interpretations of Piaget's very early work.

At the least, an acceptable stage model of illness must take into account social and cultural factors and experience, how different explanations of illness reflect different operational processes, and how the transition from one stage to another occurs.

An alternative approach is to acknowledge the criticisms that have been made of stage theory generally, and seriously consider other views of developmental processes. While specific details of other approaches differ, they share an assumption that children are active processors of information, and that a key difference between child and adult functioning is related to differences in experience (Nelson, 1986; Carey, 1985). Carey (1985) argues that children's beliefs about issues (such as how the body works) do not develop in isolation, but are part of more extensive changes in fundamental biological knowledge. Workers within the 'stage' tradition have tended to consider concepts (of health, illness, the body, death, etc.) in isolation, and have not considered how knowledge in any one domain influences knowledge in another.

In the past, the lack of any coherent theoretical framework to explain changes in children's beliefs about health and illness issues has resulted in a plethora of descriptive studies, which have yielded little in the way of prediction regarding illness behaviour, such as compliance with medical advice or preparedness to report symptoms. A satisfactory model needs to take into account the extent of vicarious learning about illness that takes place in the pre-school years. In addition, a model of illness beliefs cannot be restricted to a cognitive model, based on children's understanding of the cause of illness, but needs to be integrated within social and cultural frameworks that take account of illness-related behaviours and attitudes.

The psychological effects of chronic disease on the child

A central concern for both clinicians and researchers relates to the extent to which chronic disease influences child adjustment. Given the potential restrictions of childhood disease, it is perhaps to be expected that some adverse repercussions would occur, and that this would be reflected in deficits in intellectual, personal and social functioning. The bulk of research suggests that some deficits can occur in all these areas. However, differences in constitution of the samples, methods of outcome assessment, and source of information have all contributed to inconsistencies in the research literature.

Chronic disease: a single diagnosis?

This book is about coping with chronic childhood disease. To the extent that all chronic diseases are associated with emotional demands and practical difficulties, create restrictions for the child and family and require them to develop effective coping strategies, this approach seems to be justified. It can be further justified if it is remembered that many chronic diseases are rare, and affect relatively small numbers of children. The psychological needs of any single disease group may be under-estimated or dismissed, because they are too small to be an effective lobby. This may be of practical significance, when it comes to pressing for resources at home or school –

it may be more persuasive to demand additional resources for all chronically sick children and their families rather than for isolated cases. In research, this 'non-categorical' approach, that care-taking and emotional demands of chronic disease in general are more important than idiosyncratic details of particular conditions, is reflected in epidemiological work (see Pless & Roghmann, 1971; Rutter, Graham & Yule, 1970; Cadman, Boyle, Szatmari & Offord, 1987).

However, epidemiological surveys have indicated that some features of disease increase the relative risk of maladjustment in the child. Gross indicators include CNS dysfunction or physical disability. An alternative approach is in fact to place greater emphasis on the unique characteristics and limitations of a particular disease. Lipowski (1971), for example, argued that diseases differed in the extent to which they threatened the child's life, mobility or social and intellectual functioning. Later work has refined and elaborated this descriptive framework; diseases differ in severity, visibility, reversibility and the amount and type of care demanded of child and parents.

Methodologically, this latter approach is characterised by small-scale, clinic-based studies, where the implications of a single disease are explored in relation to a wide range of outcome variables. The disadvantage of this method is that results may reflect idiosyncracies of a particular clinic and its management, or specific population characteristics, and not be readily generalisable to all children suffering from that particular condition. This approach may be criticised in that significant over-estimation (or indeed under-estimation) of difficulties may occur, because of the make-up of the particular clinic sample.

It is unfortunate that researchers tend to be committed to one or other of these extreme positions. Undoubtedly, chronic disease is a 'risk' factor, but it is necessary to develop theory-based predictions about which features of a disease expose a child to significantly greater risk, and if, indeed, some features actually operate to modify the adverse effects. (For example, it has been suggested that children with asthma who are unable to participate in games and physical activities spend more time in sedentary occupations and in the company of adults, resulting in heightened learning and concentration skills.)

It has become clear that single variables such as severity do not determine adjustment in a simple, linear fashion. Although some research suggests that maladjustment increases with severity, other research finds the opposite relationship, and still other work reports a curvilinear effect, such that least maladjustment occurs for children with the mildest and most severe forms of a single disease. The measurement of severity is, in any case, far more difficult than was originally supposed. There are usually a number of objective measures for any single disease, and much work suggests that subjective estimates, based on a family's perceptions of disease limitations, are more critical.

The search for individual disease parameters which predict maladjustment is doubtless idealistic. Diseases vary simultaneously along many dimensions, which makes it impossible to conduct well-controlled studies. Undoubtedly, individuals differ in their appraisal of the demands of a given disease. Some children, who dislike physical activity enormously, may feel a great relief that they are excused from the afternoon's cross-country run. For other children, this same limitation can be devastating. Some mothers have far greater difficulty in keeping the house dust-free, while others take domestic work in their stride. Much greater account needs to be taken of the individual's appraisal of the restrictions and demands of disease and treatment.

Outcome measures

The impact of chronic disease on a child's adjustment has traditionally been measured in terms of (a) IQ, achievement test scores and school attendance; (b) 'social' variables, such as participation in social or sporting activities and friendship patterns; and (c) personality variables, including temperament, hostility, aggression, depression or self-esteem. Some of these measures have been selected more for their apparent objectivity than their theoretical relevance to the child's adjustment. In no case is this criticism more justified than with respect to IQ.

Intelligence

With few exceptions (such as children suffering from some kinds of epilepsy or other diseases which are known to affect the CNS), there is little reason to suppose that IQ will be affected by chronic disease. Most clinicians are not aware of the variability that can occur in IQ scores as a result of tester-style or day-to-day fluctuations in the child's health and motivation. This has resulted in unreasonable faith being placed in the IQ score, with decisions taken about the child's education which are unfounded. Neither is IQ the most appropriate outcome measure to assess the effects of interventions or treatment protocols. IQ scores have formed the basis of evaluation programmes concerned with the effects of radiation and chemotherapy on children with leukaemia, and in assessing the effects of diet on children with phenylketonuria. However, IQ tests are not sufficiently sensitive to detect early or subtle defects in ability; either do they indicate the child's level of functioning outside the traditional classroom setting. Less emphasis needs to be placed on IQ scores, and more on the effects of chronic disease on the child's social competence and learning potential. There is little indication that IQ scores are susceptible to change as a function of teaching, while social competence and adaptation can be enhanced quite successfully. Assessment of the limitations of chronic disease should be made with respect to the child's competent functioning in a wide range of situations, and not be restricted to a score on an IQ or achievement test.

In any case, researchers have done little more than to speculate about the processes whereby IQ (or any other indicator) can be compromised. It is not clear whether chronic disease acts cumulatively, progressively limiting the child's learning. An equally plausible hypothesis is that chronic disease limits the child's ability to acquire a particular skill or set of skills, and subsequent learning is impeded because the child is unable to build on more fundamental learning. The processes whereby development is compromised are important, both theoretically and in terms of practical implications for remediation.

Social development

It was noted in Chapter 4 that older children and adolescents with chronic disease were more restricted in their social activities than healthy peers, and more restricted than younger children with chronic disease. Researchers have invariably been content to describe such limitations, and not consider their implications: what follows from this kind of disadvantage? Friendships provide children with optimal environments for learning cooperative skills and developing the basis for later more intimate relationships. Although there are suggestions that children with chronic disease lack friends, there is little real indication that they are actively disliked or avoided. (However, Tin and Teasdale (1985) found that children with spina bifida were avoided in the playground.)

Social rejection is clearly associated with problems in later life

(Parker & Asher, 1987). For this reason, it is insufficient to hint that children with chronic disease have difficulties with peer relationships, without clarifying their nature or extent, and considering the long-term implications. There are suggestions, too, that children who lack friends have less sophisticated ideas about the reciprocities and intimacies involved in friendship (Selman, 1980). Future work needs to consider the meaning of friendship to children with chronic disease, rather than rely exclusively on measures of participation in social activities.

There are also questions about the meaning of friendships with healthy children compared with friendships based on the shared experience of chronic disease. The extent to which children choose friendships independently of, or based on, chronic disease, may well have important implications for self-definition.

Personality

Standardised measures of personality are not always the most appropriate for work with groups of children with chronic disease, especially where these were developed primarily for use with psychiatric samples. Often these measures contain items which have different meanings for children with chronic disease. Measures of depression, for example, often include several somatic items. Heiligstein and Jacobson (1988) found that depression (as measured by the Children's Depression rating scale) was significantly associated with functional impairment amongst children and adolescents with cancer. Removal of the somatic items from the depression scale yielded a measure which was not correlated with functional impairment, but did correlate with clinical judgement. Since disease is inevitably associated with increased fatigue or irritability, the child's score is inflated, and the conclusion likely to be drawn that the child is depressed. Standardised measures need to be given careful scrutiny to ensure that inappropriate items are excluded. Alternatively, more measures which are developed for chronic disease groups need to be available.

Other issues in child adjustment research

Time

Most research has been restricted to cross-sectional studies including children with a given disease but at an unspecified stage of treatment.

Work with those with leukaemia usually specifies whether the children are well and in remission contrasted with those in relapse, but other studies do little more than state the mean time since diagnosis for the group as a whole. Consequently, much research is based on groups of children who vary in terms of the time since diagnosis, from several weeks to many years. Such a design does not enable a distinction to be made as to whether difficulties occur on diagnosis and subsequently become less important, or whether difficulties become increasingly exaggerated as the time since diagnosis increases. Either hypothesis may be intuitively acceptable.

Neither has there been much interest in the long-term effects of chronic disease. Such research as there is suggests that the effects of chronic disease may be irreversible. For example, young adults who had been successfully treated for leukaemia continued to show deficits in psychosocial functioning (Mulhern, Wasserman, Friedman & Fairclough, 1989). Fritz and Williams (1988) found that survivors of childhood cancer continued to have concerns about their bodies, as well as anxieties about their sexuality, attractiveness and reproductive capacity. As treatment for chronic disease becomes more successful (in terms of extending life-expectancy), greater attention needs to be paid to the conflicts and dilemmas which are created for the survivors. Many patients need assurance that the disease is not inheritable, otherwise they will choose not to have children in order to safeguard their own health, and that of their offspring (Holmes & Holmes, 1975).

Gender

Males are physically more vulnerable than females (for a review, see Gualtieri & Hicks, 1985). Despite this well-documented finding, little attempt has been made to investigate the differential vulnerability of boys and girls to chronic disease. Data that are available suggest that boys show more adverse psychological responses than girls (Hurtig & White, 1986).

It is possible that parents treat chronically sick boys and girls differently: traditionally parents are more nurturing towards girls than boys (Whiting & Edwards, 1988). The potential effects of disease combined with differences in parental responses may well mean that the implications of chronic disease are not the same for both genders. It is surprising, given the well-established fact of heightened male vulnerability, that more care has not been taken in examining the differential effects of chronic disease.

Adjustment in families

Chronic disease has been described as a diagnosis which affects the whole family. Certainly, it is difficult to imagine that any individual involved with a child with chronic disease could be immune from its repercussions. Research has tended to focus, first, on identifying the differential properties of various diseases, to assess whether some conditions impose more demanding burdens than others. Perhaps the most recent work in this tradition is that of Varni and Wallander (1988) and their colleagues, who have attempted to identify the 'functional care demands' inherent in various conditions. Again, however, it must be stressed that there are no absolute measures of such demands, and families vary widely in their subjective appraisal of care-taking tasks.

A second approach has been to look at characteristics of families, especially in terms of practical, economic and psychological resources, the educational level of parents and their inter-relationships and communication patterns. There is a danger in this approach that families will be dichotomised into 'good' and 'poor' copers, based on an underlying assumption that these are stable attributes of families, and immutable to change. Little attention has been paid to changes in family coping as a function of time since the child was diagnosed, changes in the child's physical health, or additional crises that the family may confront. Neither has consideration been given to the fact that family relationships change and develop over time, whether or not a child has a chronic disease.

As children develop, they elicit different emotional responses from care-takers. While mothers' involvement with young children takes the form of concrete and practical guidance, they increasingly rely on verbal instructions as the child gets older (Heckhausen, 1987). During middle-childhood, the mother–child relationship moves to a more equal partnership, with both mother and child accepting that the child's behaviour can be self-regulated, within mutually agreed limits (Maccoby, 1984). The amount of physical contact decreases as the child increases in size. Changes continue into adolescence. However, these are not necessarily characterised by detachment, turmoil and termination, and many adolescents report enjoying joint activities with their parents during this period (Collins & Russell, 1988).

Research concerned with the effects of a child's chronic disease on families has been divorced from this natural background. The focus has been rather narrowly on mother–child relationships, with little acknowledgement made of the natural developments which occur in family dynamics. There is also an assumption that development occurs exclusively in the child. In fact, development takes place for all family members, albeit more slowly in the adults. Younger mothers have more difficulties in dealing with disruptive behaviour in their children, and setting appropriate limits. Walter (1986) suggests that women at different stages of development bring their own expectations to child-rearing and varied social skills to deal with the family environment. Again, research has tended to consider all mothers of children with chronic disease as a homogeneous group, taking no account of variables such as these which have been shown to influence normal family functioning.

These arguments apply equally to considerations of the father–child relationship. Fathers appear to fulfil different needs for their children compared with mothers, but the relationship should not be considered as any less close. It is essential that the role of fathers in rearing a chronically sick child comes under closer research scrutiny. At the same time, this work needs to be integrated with the rapidly expanding body of knowledge considering the role of fathers in child-rearing generally. The importance of fathers is in the degree to which their behaviour does not duplicate that of the mother, and in the degree to which they support maternal caregiving rather than replicate it.

For all parents, raising their children can be highly demanding, and sometimes tedious. They are confronted by a series of situations in which complex decisions are required. Idealistic views on parent-ing and the realities of the situation must be reconciled, and concrete decisions made about discipline and the manner in which parents effect control. Parents of chronically sick children face the same dilemmas, with the added burden of reconciling the family activities within limits imposed by the disease. To this end, they are families coping with very special circumstances, rather than pathological or deviant ones.

Psychology–paediatric liaison

Progress in understanding the psychological effects of chronic disease has been determined, and to some extent limited, by theoreti-cal models and interventions handed down from adult health psychology. These approaches have some merit, but do not always address problems which are specific to the context in which child development occurs. There has been a failure to integrate the work within a developmental framework. Research questions have centred on the impact of chronic disease, without acknowledging the interdependence between adjustment to disease and general developmental processes.

Secondly, the impact of research work is limited by the ability of psychologists to communicate the findings to paediatricians and parents, ensuring that 'practical implications' are both viable and implemented.

Psychological work is in fact dependent on paediatric appraisal if it is to take place at all. It is necessary to obtain paediatric approval before research can begin, and patient participation can be influenced dramatically by the extent to which paediatricians are prepared to encourage patients and endorse the potential value of the research. Paediatrician involvement can be limited to this approval-giving status, in which case psychologists must educate themselves about the nature of disease and its treatment, and make their own decisions as to the implications of the work for clinical practice.

Alternatively, paediatricians and psychologists can work more closely to delineate problem areas. In this case, the paediatrician brings a great deal of knowledge and expertise about disease and management, while the psychologist may be in a better position to identify potential difficulties for the child, as well as contributing a body of knowledge about research design and measurement techniques. Effective research, which is methodologically sound and clinically relevant, requires such a collaborative model of psychologist—paediatrician involvement.

The potential pit-falls in this relationship have recently received considerable attention, at least in books and reviews directed at psychologists (Drotar, 1989; Stabler, 1988). Differences in training and background, preferences for different kinds of research methods and lack of awareness about what other specialties can (and cannot) offer, can be so pronounced that effective collaboration is curtailed. These difficulties are only likely to be lessened by more integrated training programmes and joint dissemination of research findings which are equally accessible to both disciplines. I hope this book can make some contribution to bridging the gap between research and clinical practice.

References

Abbott, N. C., Hansen, P. & Lewis, K. (1970). Dress rehearsal for the hospital. *American Journal of Nursing*, **70**, 2360.

Abu-Saad, H. (1984). Cultural group indicators of pain in children. *Children's Health Care*, **13**, 11–14.

Achenbach, T. & Edelbrook, C. (1983). *Manual for the Child Behavior Checklist and Revised Child Behavior Profile*. Burlington: University of Vermont.

Ack, M., Miller, I. & Weil, W. B. (1961). Intelligence of children with diabetes mellitus. *Pediatrics*, **25**, 764–70.

Acosta, P. B., Fiedler, J. L. & Koch, R. (1968). Mothers' dietary management of PKU children. *Journal of the American Dietetic Association*, **53**, 460–4.

Aisenberg, R. B., Wolff, P. H., Rosenthal, A. & Nadas, A. S. (1973). Psychological impact of cardiac catheterization. *Pediatrics*, **51**, 1051–9.

Alexander, A. B. (1983). The nature of asthma. In P. J. McGrath & P. Firestone (eds.), *Pediatrics and Adolescent Behavioral Medicine: Issues in Treatment*. New York: Springer.

Allen, D. A., Affleck, G., Tennen, H., McGrade, B. J. & Ratzan, S. (1984). Concerns of children with a chronic illness: a cognitive-developmental study of juvenile diabetes. *Child: Care, Health and Development*, **10**, 211–18.

Allen, L. & Zigler, E. (1986). Psychological adjustment of seriously ill children. *Journal of the American Academy of Child and Adolescent Psychiatry*, **25**, 708–12.

Altschuler, A. (1974). Books that help children deal with a hospital experience. DHEW Publication No. HSA 74-5402. Washington, DC; US Government Printing Office.

Anderson, B. J., Hagen, J., Barclay, C., Goldstein, G., Kandt, R. & Bacon, G. (1984). Cognitive and school performance in diabetic children (Abstract). *Diabetes*, **33** (Suppl. 1), 21A.

Anderson, H. R., Bailey, P. A., Cooper, J. A., Palmer, J. S. & West, S. (1983). Morbidity and school absence caused by asthma and wheezing illness. *Archives of Disease in Childhood*, **58**, 777–84.

Andrasik, F., Burke, E. J., Attanasio, V. & Rosenblum, E. L. (1985). Child, parent and physician reports of a child's headache pain: Relationships prior to and following treatment. *Headache*, **25**, 421–5.

Anhsjo, S., Humble, Y., Larsson, G., Settergren-Carlsson, G. & Sterky, G. (1981). Personality changes and social adjustment during the first three years of diabetes in children. *Acta Paediatrica Scandinavia Supplement*, **70**, 321–7.

Argyris, C. (1968). Conditions for competence acquisition and theory. *Journal of Applied Behavioral Science*, **4**, 147–77.

Armstrong, R. W., Rosenbaum, P. L. & King, S. M. (1987). A randomized controlled trial of a 'buddy' programme to improve children's attitudes toward the disabled. *Developmental Medicine and Child Neurology*, **29**, 327–36.

Azarnoff, P. & Woody, P. (1981). Preparation of children for hospitalization in acute care hospitals in the United States. *Pediatrics*, **69** (3), 361–8.

Bakwin, H. & Bakwin, R. (1948). The child with asthma. *Journal of Pediatrics*, **32**, 320–3.

Baluk, U. & O'Neill, P. (1980). Health professionals' perceptions of the psychological consequences of abortion. *American Journal of Community Psychology*, **8**, 67–75.

Band, E. & Weisz, J. R. (1988). How to feel better when it feels bad: Children's perspectives on coping with everyday stress. *Developmental Psychology*, **24**, 247–53.

Bane, M. J. (1976). *Here to stay: American Families in the Twentieth Century*. New York: Basic.

Banion, J. R., Miles, M. S. & Carter, M. C. (1983). Problems of mothers in management of children with diabetes. *Diabetes Care*, **6**, 548–51.

Barr, R. (1983). Variations on the theme of pain: 28A Pain tolerance and developmental change in pain perception. In M. D. Levine, W. B. Carey, A. C. Crocker & R. T. Gross (eds.), *Developmental Behavioral Pediatrics*. Philadelphia, PA: Saunders, pp. 505–12.

Barrios, B., Hartman, D. & Shigetomi, C. (1981). Fears and anxieties in children. In E. J. Mash & L. G. Terdal (eds.), *Behavioral Assessment of Childhood Disorders*. New York: Guilford Press.

Barrios, B. A. & Shigetomi, C. C. (1980). Coping-skills training: Potential for the prevention of fears and anxieties. *Behavior Therapy*, **11**, 431–9.

Baum, J. D. (1981). Home monitoring of diabetic control. *Archives of Disease in Childhood*, **56**, 897–9.

Beales, J. G., Holt, P. J. L., Keen, J. H. & Mellor, V. P. (1983). Children with juvenile chronic arthritis: Their beliefs about their illness and therapy. *Annals of the Rheumatic Diseases*, **42**, 481–6.

Beck, A. L., Nethercut, G. E., Crittenden, M. R. & Hewins, J. (1986). Visibility of handicap, self-concept, and social maturity among young adult survivors of end-stage renal disease. *Developmental and Behavioral Pediatrics*, **7**, 93–6.

Bernstein, A. C. & Cowan, P. A. (1981). Children's conceptions of birth and sexuality. In R. Bibace & M. E. Walsh (eds.), *New Directions for Child Development: No. 14. Children's Conceptions of Health, Illness and Bodily Functions*. San Francisco: Jossey Bass, pp. 9–30.

Beyer, J. E. (1984). *The Oucher: A User's Manual and Technical Report*. Evanston, IL: The Hospital Play Equipment Co.

Bibace, R. & Walsh, M. E. (eds.) (1981). Children's conceptions of illness. In R. Bibace & M. E. Walsh (eds.), *New Directions for Child Development: No. 14. Children's Conceptions of Health, Illness and Bodily Functions*. San Francisco: Jossey Bass.

Billings, A. G., Moos, R. H., Miller, J. J. III & Gottlieb, J. E. (1987). Psychosocial adaptation in juvenile rheumatic disease: A controlled evaluation. *Health Psychology*, **6**, 343–59.

Binger, C., Ablin, A., Feuerstein, R., Kushner, J., Zoger, S. & Mikkelsen, C. (1969). Childhood leukemia: Emotional impact on patient and family. *New England Journal of Medicine*, **280**, 414–18.

Birleson, P., Hudson, I., Buchanan, D. G. & Wolff, S. (1987). Clinical evaluation of a self-rating scale for depressive disorder in childhood (depression self-rating scale). *Journal of Child Psychology and Psychiatry*, **28**, 43–60.

Blos, P. (1978). Children think about illness: Their conceptual beliefs. In E. Gellert (ed.), *Psychosocial Aspects of Pediatric Care*. New York: Grune & Stratton, pp. 1–17.

Blotcky, A. D., Raczynski, J. M., Gurwich, R. & Smith, K. (1985). Family influences on hopelessness among children early in the cancer experience. *Journal of Pediatric Psychology*, **10**, 479–94.

Bluebond-Langner, M. (1978). *The Private World of Dying Children*. Princeton: Princeton University Press.

Boll, T. J., Domino, E. & Mattson, A. E. (1978). Parenting attitudes: The role of personality style and childhood long-term illnesses. *Journal of Psychosomatic Research*, **22**, 209–13.

Bolstad, C. H. (1975). A behavioral comparison of handicapped and normal children within the family. *Dissertation Abstracts International*, **35**, 4160B.

Borner, A. & Steinhausen, H. C. (1977). A psychological study of family characteristics in juvenile diabetes. *Pediatric and Adolescent Endocrinology*, **3**, 36–51.

Botvin, G. J. (1983). Prevention of adolescent substance abuse through the development of personal and social competence. In T. Glynn and C. Leukeveld (eds.), *Preventing Adolescent Drug Abuse: Intervention Strategies*. DHSS Publication No. (ADM) 83-128. Washington, DC: US Government Printing Office.

Botvin, G. J. & Wills, T. A. (1985). Personal and social skills training: Cognitive-behavioral approaches to substance abuse prevention. In C. S. Bell & R. Battjes (eds.), *Prevention Research: Deterring Drug Abuse Among Children and Adolescents*. National Institute on Drug Abuse

Research Monograph 63. DHSS Publication No. (AOM) 85-1334. Washington, DC: Superintendent of Documents, US Government Printing Office, pp. 8–49.

Bowlby, J. (1960). Separation anxiety. *International Journal of Psychoanalysis*, **41**, 89–113.

(1980). *Attachment and Loss: Vol. 3. Sadness and Depression*. New York: Basic Books.

Bradbury, J. A. & Smith, C. W. (1983). An assessment of the diabetic knowledge of school teachers. *Archives of Disease in Childhood*, **58**, 692–6.

Breslau, N. (1982). Siblings of disabled children: Birth order and age-spacing effects. *Journal of Abnormal Child Psychology*, **10**, 85–96.

(1983). Care of disabled children and women's time use. *Medical Care*, **21**, 620–9.

Breslau, N. & Marshall, I. A. (1985). Psychological disturbance in children with physical disabilities: Continuity and change in a 5-year follow-up. *Journal of Abnormal Child Psychology*, **13**, 199–216.

Breslau, N., Salkever, D. & Staruch, K. S. (1982). Women's labor force activity and responsibility for disabled dependents. *Journal of Health and Social Behavior*, **67**, 344–53.

Breslau, N., Staruch, K. S. & Mortimer, E. A. (1982). Psychological distress in mothers of disabled children. *American Journal of Diseases in Children*, **136**, 682–6.

Breslau, N., Weitzman, M. & Messenger, K. (1981). Psychological functioning of siblings of disabled children. *Pediatrics*, **67**, 344–53.

Brett, A. (1983). Preparing children for hospitalization – a classroom teaching approach. *Journal of School Health*, **53**, 561–3.

Brewster, A. B. (1982). Chronically ill hospitalized children's concepts of their illness. *Pediatrics*, **69**, 355–62.

Brody, G. H. & Stoneman, Z. (1983). Children with atypical siblings: socialization outcomes and clinical practice. In B. B. Lahey & A. E. Kazdin (eds.), *Advances in Clinical Child Psychology*. New York: Plenum Press, pp. 285–301.

Brown, A. L. & De Loache, J. S. (1978). Skills, plans and self-regulation. In R. Siegler (ed.), *Children's Thinking; What Develops?* Hillsdale, NJ: Erlbaum.

Brown, J. M., O'Keeffe, J., Sanders, S. H. & Baker, B. (1986). Developmental changes in children's cognition to stressful and painful situations. *Journal of Pediatric Psychology*, **11**, 343–57.

Bruhn, J. G., Hampton, J. W. & Chandler, B. C. (1971). Clinical marginality and psychological adjustment in hemophilia. *Journal of Psychosomatic Research*, **15**, 207–13.

Burbach, D. J. & Peterson, L. (1986). Children's concepts of physical illness: A review and critique of the cognitive-developmental literature. *Health Psychology*, **5**, 307–25.

Burr, C. K. (1985). Impact on the family of a chronically ill child. In N. Hobbs & J. M. Perrin (eds.), *Issues in the Care of Children with Chronic Illness*. San Francisco: Jossey Bass, pp. 24–40.

Bush, J. P., Melamed, B. G., Sheras, P. J. & Greenbaum, P. E. (1986). Mother–child patterns of coping with anticipatory medical stress. *Health Psychology*, **5**, 137–57.

Cadman, D., Boyle, M., Szatmari, P. & Offord, D. R. (1987). Chronic illness, disability, and mental and social well-being: Findings of the Ontario Child Health Study. *Pediatrics*, **79**, 705–12.

Caldwell, H. S., Leveque, K. L. & Lane, D. M. (1974). Group psychotherapy in the management of hemophilia. *Psychological Reports*, **35**, 339–42.

Califano, J. A. Jnr. (1979). *Healthy People: The Surgeon General's Report on Health Promotion and Disease Prevention*. Washington, DC: US Government Printing Office.

Carey, S. (1985). *Conceptual Change in Childhood*. Massachusetts: MIT.

Carver, C. S., Scheier, M. F. & Weintraub, J. M. (1989). Assessing coping strategies: A theoretically based approach. *Journal of Personality and Social Psychology*, **56**, 267–83.

Cassell, S. (1965). Effect of brief puppet-therapy upon the emotional responses of children undergoing cardiac catheterization. *Journal of Counselling Psychology*, **29**, 1–8.

Cassell, S. & Paul, M. (1967). The role of puppet therapy on the emotional responses of children hospitalized for cardiac catheterization. *Pediatrics*, **71**, 233–9.

Chan, J. M. (1980). Preparation for procedures and surgery through play. *Paediatrician*, **9**, 210–19.

Chesler, M. A. (1984). Support systems for parents of children with cancer. Paper presented at the American Cancer Society Conference on Human Values and Cancer, New York.

Chesler, M. A., Paris, J. & Barbarin, O. A. (1986). 'Telling' the child with cancer: Parental choices to share information with ill children. *Journal of Pediatric Psychology*, **11**, 497–516.

Chess, S. & Thomas, A. (1986). *Temperament in Clinical Practice*. New York: Guilford.

Chi, M. T. H., Glaser, R. & Rees, E. (1982). Expertise in problem-solving. In R. Sternberg (ed.), *Advances in the Psychology of Human Intelligence*, Vol. I. Hillsdale, NJ: Lawrence Erlbaum.

Chodoff, P., Friedman, S. & Hamburg, D. A. (1964). Stress, defences, and coping behavior: Observation in parents of children with malignant disease. *American Journal of Psychiatry*, **120**, 743–9.

Claerhout, S. & Lutzker, J. R. (1981). Increasing children's self-initiated compliance to dental regimes. *Behavior Therapy*, **12**, 165–76.

Clarson, C., Daneman, D., Frank, M., Link, J., Perlman, K. & Erhlich, R. M. (1985). Self-monitoring of blood glucose: How accurate are children with diabetes at reading chemstrip bG? *Diabetes Care*, **8**, 354–8.

Close, H., Davies, A. G., Price, D. A. & Goodyer, I. M. (1986). Emotional difficulties in diabetes mellitus. *Archives of Disease in Childhood*, **61**, 337–40.

Clunies-Ross, C. & Lansdown, R. (1988). Concepts of death, illness and isolation found in children with leukaemia. *Child: Care, Health and Development*, **14**, 373–86.

Colby, A., Kohlberg, L., Candee, D., Gibbs, J., Hewer, A., Kauffman, K., Power, C. & Speicher-Dubin, B. (1990). *Assessing Moral Judgements: A Manual*. New York: Cambridge University Press (in press).

Collier, G. & Etzwiler, D. (1971). Comparative study of diabetes knowledge among juvenile diabetics and their parents. *Diabetes*, **20**, 51–7.

Collins, W. A. & Russell, G. (1988). Mother–child and father–child relationships in middle childhood and adolescence. Cited in Hartup, W. W. (1989). Social relationships and their developmental significance. *American Psychologist*, **44**, 120–6.

Compas, B. E. (1987). Coping with stress during childhood and adolescence. *Psychological Bulletin*, **101**, 393–403.

Compas, B. E., Malcarne, V. L. & Fondacaro, K. M. (1988). Coping with stressful events in older children and young adolescents. *Journal of Consulting and Clinical Psychology*, **56**, 405–11.

Connell, D. B., Turner, R. R. & Mason, E. F. (1985). Summary of findings of the School Health Education Evaluation. Health promotion effectiveness, implementation and costs. *Journal of School Health*, **55**, 316–21.

Consumers Association (1980). *Children in Hospital*. London: Consumers Association.

Cousens, P., Waters, B., Said, J. & Stevens, M. (1988). Cognitive effects of cranial irradiation in leukaemia: a survey and meta-analysis. *Journal of Child Psychology and Psychiatry*, **29**, 839–52.

Craig, K. J. D., McMahon, R. J., Morison, J. D. & Zaskow, C. (1984). Developmental changes in infant pain expression during immunization injections. *Social Science and Medicine*, **19**, 1331–7.

Crain, A., Sussman, M. & Weill, W. Jr. (1966). Effects of a diabetic child on marital integration and related measures of family functioning. *Journal of Health and Human Behavior*, **7**, 122–7.

Creer, T. L., Harm, D. L. & Marion, R. J. (1988). Childhood asthma. In D. Routh (ed.), *Handbook of Pediatric Psychology*. New York: Guilford Press, pp. 162–89.

Creer, T. & Leung, P. (1981). The development and evaluation of a self-management program for children with asthma. In *Self-Management Educational Programs for Childhood Asthma*, Vol. 2. Bethesda, MA: National Institute of Allergy and Infectious Diseases, pp. 107–28.

Crider, C. (1981). Children's conceptions of the body interior. In R. Bibace & M. E. Walsh (eds.), *New Directions for Child Development: No. 14. Children's Conceptions of Health, Illness and Bodily Functions*. San Francisco: Jossey Bass, pp. 49–66.

Crittenden, M. & Gofman, H. (1976). Follow-ups and downs: The medical center, the family, and the school. *Journal of Pediatric Psychology*, **1**, 66–8.

Crocker, A. (1981). The involvement of siblings of children with handicaps. In A. Milunsky (ed.), *Coping with Crisis and Handicap*. New York: Plenum.

Crocker, E. (1979). Hospital books for children. *Canadian Nurse*, **75**, 33.

Crowl, M. (1980). Case study: The basic process of art therapy as demonstrated by efforts to allay a child's fear of surgery. *American Journal of Art Therapy*, **19**, 49–51.

Dahl, R. (1986). *Boy: Tales of Childhood*. Middlesex, England: Puffin Books.

Daneman, D., Siminerio, L., Transne, D., Betschart, J., Drash, A. & Becker, D. (1985). The role of self-monitoring of blood-glucose in the routine managements of children with insulin-dependent diabetes mellitus. *Diabetes Care*, **8**, 1–4.

Daniels, D., Miller, J. J., Billings, A. H. & Moos, R. H. (1986). Psychosocial functioning of siblings of children with rheumatic disease. *Journal of Pediatrics*, **109**, 379–83.

Debuskey, M. (1970). Orchestration of care. In M. Debuskey (ed.), *The Chronically Ill Child and his Family*. Springfield, Illinois: Thomas.

Dorner, S. (1976). Adolescents with spina bifida: How they see their situation. *Archives of Disease in Childhood*, **51**, 439–44.

Douglas, J. (1975). Early hospital admissions and later disturbances of behaviour and learning. *Developmental Medicine and Child Neurology*, **17**, 456–80.

Drotar, D. (1989). Psychological research in pediatric settings: Lessons from the field. *Journal of Pediatric Psychology*, **14**, 63–74.

Drotar, D. & Crawford, P. (1985). Psychological adaptation of siblings of chronically ill children: Research and practice implications. *Developmental and Behavioral Pediatrics*, **6**, 355–62.

Drotar, D., Crawford, P. & Ganofsky, M. A. (1984). Prevention with chronically ill children. In M. Roberts & L. Peterson (eds.), *Prevention of Problems in Childhood*. New York: Wiley, pp. 232–65.

Duffy, E. (1962). *Activation of all Behavior*. New York: Wiley.

Dunbar, J. & Stunkard, A. J. (1977). Adherence to diet and drug regimen. In R. Levy, R. Rifkind, B. Dennis & N. Ernst (eds.), *Nutrition, Lipids, and Coronary Heart Disease*. New York: Raven Press.

Dunn, J. (1987). Introduction. In F. F. Schachter & R. K. Stone (eds.), Practical concerns about siblings: Bridging the research-practice gap. *Journal of Children in Contemporary Society*, **19**, 1–11.

(1988). Sibling influences on childhood development. *Journal of Child Psychology and Psychiatry*, **29**, 119–28.

Dweck, C. S., Guetz, T. E. & Strauss, N. L. (1980). Sex differences in learned helplessness: IV. An experimental and naturalistic study of failure generalization and its mediators. *Journal of Personality and Social Psychology*, **38**, 441–52.

Dweck, C. S. & Licht, B. G. (1980). Learned helplessness and intellectual achievement. In J. Garber & M. E. P. Sehgman (eds.), *Human Helplessness: Theory and Applications*. New York: Academic Press, pp. 197–221.

Dweck, C. S. & Reppucci, N. D. (1973). Learned helplessness and reinforcement responsibility in children. *Journal of Personality and Social Psychology*, **25**, 109–16.

Dweck, C. S. & Wortman, C. B. (1982). Learned helplessness, anxiety, and achievement motivation: Neglected parallels in cognition, affective and coping responses. In H. W. Krohne & L. Laux (eds.), *Achievements, Stress and Anxiety*. Washington, DC: Hemisphere, pp. 93–125.

Easson, W. (1970). *The Dying Child: The Management of the Child or Adolescent who is Dying*. Springfield, Illinois: Thomas.

Eiser, C. (1980). How leukaemia affects a child's schooling. *British Journal of Social and Clinical Psychology*, **19**, 365–8.

(1984). Communicating with sick and hospitalized children. *Journal of Child Psychology and Psychiatry*, **24**, 181–9.

(1985). *The Psychology of Childhood Illness*. New York: Springer-Verlag.

(1986). Effects of chronic illness on the child's intellectual development. *Journal of the Royal Society of Medicine*, **79**, 2–3.

(1987). Chronic childhood illness. In J. Orford (ed.), *Coping with Disorders in the Family*. London: Croom Helm, pp. 217–37.

(1989). Children's concepts of illness: Towards an alternative to the 'Stage' approach. *Psychology and Health*, **3**, 93–101.

Eiser, C. & Eiser, J. R. (1988). *Evaluation of 'Double Take': A Drugs Education Package*. New York: Springer.

Eiser, C., Eiser, J. R. & Hunt, J. (1986). Comprehension of metaphysical explanations of illness. *Early Child Development and Care*, **26**, 79–88.

Eiser, C., Eiser, J. R. & Lang, J. (1989). Scripts in children's reports of medical events. *European Journal of the Psychology of Education*, **4**, 377–84.

Eiser, C. & Hanson, L. (1989). Preparing children for hospital: A school-based intervention. *The Professional Nurse*, **4**, 297–300.

Eiser, C. & Patterson, D. (1983). Children's perception of hospital: A preliminary study. *International Journal of Nursing Studies* (1984), **21**, 45–50.

Eiser, C., Patterson, D. & Town, R. (1985). Knowledge of diabetes and implications for self-care. *Diabetic Medicine*, **2**, 288–91.

Eiser, C. & Town, C. (1987). Teachers' concerns about chronically sick children. Implications for paediatricians. *Developmental Medicine and Child Neurology*, **29**, 56–63.

Eiser, C., Town, C. & Tripp, J. H. (1988). Knowledge and understanding of asthma. *Child: Care, Health and Development*, **14**, 11–24.

Elkins, P. D. & Roberts, M. C. (1983). Psychosocial preparation for pediatric hospitalization. *Clinical Psychology Review*, **3**, 275–95.

(1984). A preliminary evaluation of hospital preparation for nonpatient children: Primary prevention in a 'Let's pretend hospital'. *Children's Health Care*, **13**, 31–6.

(1985). Reducing medical fears in a general population of children: A comparison of three audio–visual modeling procedures. *Journal of Pediatric Psychology*, **10**, 65–75.

Ellenberg, L., Kellerman, J., Dash, J., Higgins, G. & Zeltzer, L. (1980). Use of hypnosis for multiple symptoms in an adolescent girl with leukemia. *Journal of Adolescent Health Care*, **1**, 132–6.

Elliott, C. H., Jay, S. M. & Woody, P. (1987). An observation scale for measuring children's distress during painful medical procedures. *Journal of Pediatric Psychology*, **12**, 543–52.

Erikson, E. (1964). *Childhood and Society*. New York: Norton.

Etzwiler, D. D. & Robb, J. R. (1972). Evaluation of programmed education among juvenile diabetics and their families. *Diabetes*, **21**, 967–71.

Etzwiler, D. D. & Sines, L. K. (1962). Juvenile diabetes and its management: Family, social and academic implications. *Journal of the American Medical Association*, **181**, 304–8.

Evans, A. (1968). If a child must die. *New England Journal of Medicine*, **278**, 138–42.

Ferguson, B. F. (1979). Preparing young children for hospitalization: A comparison of two methods. *Pediatrics*, **65**, 656–64.

Ferrari, M. (1984). Chronic illness: Psychosocial effects on siblings – 1. Chronically ill boys. *Journal of Child Psychology and Psychiatry*, **25**, 459–76.

Field, T. & Goldson, E. (1984). Pacifying effects of nonnutritive sucking on term and preterm neonates during heelstick procedures. *Pediatrics*, **74**, 1012–15.

Flanagan, J. (1954). The critical incident technique. *Psychological Bulletin*, **51**, 327–58.

Flay, B. R. (1985). What we know about the social influences approach to smoking prevention: Review and recommendations. In C. S. Bell & R. Battjes (eds.), *Prevention Research: Deterring Drug Abuse among Children and Adolescents*. NIDA Research. Monograph 63. A RAUS Review Report, DHSS.

Folkman, S. & Lazarus, R. S. (1980). An analysis of coping in a middle-aged community sample. *Journal of Health and Social Behaviour*, **21**, 219–39.

Folkman, S., Lazarus, R. S., Dunkel-Schetter, C., DeLongis, A. & Gruen, R. (1986). The dynamics of a stressful encounter: Cognitive appraisal, coping and encounter outcomes. *Journal of Personality and Social Psychology*, **50**, 992–1003.

Follansbee, D. J., La Greca, A. M. & Citrin, W. S. (1983). Coping skills training for adolescents with diabetes. *Diabetes*, **32**, Suppl. 1, 147 (Abstract).

Fonagny, P., Moran, G. S., Lindsay, M. K. M., Kurtz, A. B. & Brown, R. (1987). Psychological adjustment and diabetic control. *Archives of Disease in Childhood*, **62**, 1009–13.

Fowler, M., Johnson, M. & Atkinson, S. (1985). School achievement and absence in children with chronic health conditions. *Journal of Pediatrics*, **106**, 683–7.

Freund, A., Johnson, S. B., Rosenbloom, A., Alexander, B. & Hansen, C. A. (1986). Subjective symptoms, blood glucose estimation, and blood glucose concentrations in adolescents with diabetes. *Diabetes Care*, **9**, 236–43.

Fritz, G. K. & Williams, J. R. (1988). Issues of adolescent development for survivors of childhood cancer. *Journal of the American Academy of Adolescent Psychiatry*, **27**, 712.

Furman, A. E. (1970). The child's reaction to death in the family. In B. Schoenberg, A. Carr, D. Peretz & A. Kutscher (eds.), *Loss and Grief: Psychological Management in Medical Practice*. New York: Columbia University Press.

Futterman, E. & Hoffman, I. (1973). Crises and adaptation in the families of fatally ill children. In E. J. Anthony & C. Koupernick (eds.), *The child in his family: The Impact of Disease and Death*. Yearbook of the International Association for Child Psychiatry and Allied Disciplines (Vol. II). New York: Wiley.

Gaffney, A. & Dunn, E. G. (1986). Developmental aspects of children's definition of pain. *Pain*, **26**, 105–17.

(1987). Children's understanding of the causality of pain. *Pain*, **29**, 91–104.

Garmezy, N. (1983). Stressors of childhood. In N. Garmezy & M. Rutter (eds.), *Stress, Coping and Development in Children*. St Louis, MO: McGraw-Hill, pp. 43–84.

Garner, A. M. & Thompson, C. W. (1974). Factors in the management of juvenile diabetes. *Pediatric Psychology*, **2**, 6–7.

Garner, A. M., Thompson, C. W. & Partridge, J. W. (1969). Who knows best? *Diabetes Bulletin*, **45**, 3–4.

Garralda, M. E., Jameson, R. A., Reynolds, J. M. & Postlethwaite, J. R. (1988). Psychiatric adjustment in children with chronic renal failure. *Journal of Child Psychology and Psychiatry*, **29**, 79–90.

Garvey, C. & Berndt, T. R. (1977). The organization of pretend play. *Catalogue of Selected Documents in Psychology*, **7**, No. 1589.

Gath, A. (1977). The impact of an abnormal child upon the parents. *British Journal of Psychiatry*, **130**, 405–10.

Gayton, W. F., Friedman, S. B., Tavormina, J. F. & Tucker, F. (1977). Children with cystic fibrosis. I. Psychological test findings of patients, siblings and parents. *Pediatrics*, **59**, 888–94.

Gellert, E. (1962). Children's conceptions of the content and functions of the human body. *Genetic Psychology Monographs*, **65**, 293–411.

Gelman, R. & Baillargeon, R. (1983). Review of some Piagetian concepts. In J. H. Flavell & E. M. Markman (eds.), *Handbook of Child Psychology*, Vol. III: *Cognitive Development*. New York: Wiley.

Gilbert, B., Johnson, S. B., Spillar, R., McCallum, M., Silverstein, J. & Rosenbloom, A. (1982). The effects of a peer modeling film on children learning to self-inject insulin. *Behavior Therapy*, **13**, 186–93.

Glyshaw, K., Cohen, L. H. & Towbes, L. C. (1988). Coping strategies and psychological distress: Longitudinal analyses of early and middle adolescents. (Submitted).

Gochman, D. (1971). Some correlates of children's health beliefs and potential health behavior. *Journal of Health and Social Behavior*, **12**, 148–54.

Golden, M. P., Russell, B. P., Ingersoll, G. M., Gray D. L. & Humner, K. M. (1985). Management of diabetes mellitus in children younger than 5 years of age. *American Journal of Diseases of Childhood*, **139**, 448–52.

Goldstein, A. P., Sherman, M., Gershaw, N. J., Sprafkin, R. P. & Glick, B. (1978). Training agressive adolescents in prosocial behavior. *Journal of Youth and Adolescence*, **1**, 263–79.

Gortmaker, S. L. (1985). Demography of chronic childhood diseases. In N. Hobbs & J. M. Perrin (eds.), *Issues in the Care of Children with Chronic Illness*. San Francisco: Jossey-Bass.

Goslin, E. R. (1978). Hospitalization as a life-crisis for the preschool child: A critical review. *Journal of Community Health*, **3**, 321–56.

Graham, P. J., Rutter, M. L., Yule, W. & Pless, I. B. (1967). Childhood asthma: A psychosomatic disorder? Some epidemiological considerations. *British Journal of Preventive and Social Medicine*, **21**, 78–85.

Greenberg, L. W., Jewett, L. S., Gluck, R. S., Champion, L. A. A., Leikin, S. L., Altieri, M. F. & Lipnick, R. N. (1984). Giving information for a life-threatening diagnosis. *American Journal of Diseases of Children*, **138**, 649–53.

Greenberg, H. S., Kazak, A. E. & Meadows, A. T. (1989). Psychologic functioning in 8- to 16-year-old cancer survivors and their parents. *Journal of Pediatrics*, **114**, 488–93.

Greene, P. (1975). The child with leukemia in the classroom. *American Journal of Nursing*, **75**, 86–7.

Greydanus, D. E. & Hoffman, A. D. (1979). Psychological factors in diabetes mellitus: A review of the literature with emphasis on adolescence. *American Journal of Diseases of Children*, **133**, 1061–6.

Gross, A. M., Johnson, W. G., Wildman, H. E. & Mullett, M. (1981). Coping skills training with insulin-dependent preadolescent diabetics. *Child Behavior Therapy*, **3**, 141–53.

Grossman, F. K. (1972). *Brothers and Sisters of Retarded Children*. Syracuse, NY: Syracuse University Press.

Grunau, R. V. E. & Craig, K. D. (1987). Pain expression in neonates: Facial action and cry. *Pain*, **28**, 395–410.

Gualtieri, T. & Hicks, R. E. (1985). An immunoreactive theory of selective male affliction. *The Behavioral and Brain Sciences*, **8**, 427–41.

Gustafson, P. A., Kjellman, N. I. M., Ludvigsson, J. & Cederblad, M. (1987). Asthma and family interaction. *Archives of Disease in Childhood*, **62**, 258–63.

Harkavy, J., Johnson, S. B., Silverstein, J., Spillar, R., McCallum, M. &

Rosenbloom, A.(1983). Who learns what at diabetes camp? *Journals of Pediatric Psychology*, **8**, 143–53.

Harpin, V. A. & Rutter, N. (1982). Development of emotional sweating in the newborn infant. *Archives of Disease in Childhood*, **57**, 691–5.

Harter, S. (1981). The perceived competence scale for children. *Child Development*, **53**, 87–97.

Hartup, W. W. (1983). Peer relations. In P. H. Mussen & E. M. Hetherington (eds.), *Handbook of Child Psychology*, Vol. 4: *Socialization, Personality and Social Development*. New York: Wiley, pp. 103–96.

(1989). Social relationships and their developmental significance. *American Psychologist*, **44**, 120–6.

Hauser, S., Jacobson, A., Wertlieb, D., Brink, S. & Wentworth, D. (1985). The contribution of family environment to perceived competence and illness adjustment in diabetic and acutely ill adolescents. *Family Relations*, **34**, 99–108.

Hauser, S., Jacobson, A., Wertlieb, D., Weiss-Perry, B., Follansbee, D., Wolfsdorf, J. I., Herskowitz, R. D., Houlihan, J. & Rajapark, D. C. (1986). Children with recently diagnosed diabetes: Interactions within their families. *Health Psychology*, **5**, 273–96.

Hauser, S. T., Weiss, B., Follansbee, D., Powers, S., Jacobson, A., Noam, G. & Rajapark, D. C. (1985). Adolescent development and family transaction. In S. Sugerman (ed.), *Family Therapy and Individual Therapy: Critical Issues of the Interface*. Rockville, MD: Aspen Systems, pp. 84–103.

Hayden, P. W., Davenport, S. L. H. & Campbell, M. M. (1979). Adolescents with myelodysphasia: Impact of physical disability on emotional maturation. *Pediatrics*, **64**, 53–9.

Heckhausen, J. (1987). Balancing for weaknesses and challenging developmental potential: A longitudinal study of mother–infant dyads in apprenticeship interactions. *Developmental Psychology*, **23**, 762–70.

Heffernan, M. & Azarnoff, P. (1971). Factors in reducing children's anxiety about clinic visits. *Health Services and Mental Health Administration Reports*, **86**, 1131–5.

Heiligstein, E. & Jacobson, P. B. (1988). Differentiating depression in medically ill children and adolescents. *Journal of the American Academy of Adolescent Psychiatry*, **27**, 716.

Heisler, A. B. & Friedman, S. B. (1981). Social and psychological considerations in chronic disease: with particular reference to the management of seizure disorders. *Journal of Pediatric Psychology*, **6**, 239–50.

Heller, A., Rafman, S., Zvagulis, I. & Pless, I. B. (1985). Birth defects and psychosocial adjustment. *American Journal of Diseases of Children*, **139**, 257–63.

Herz, E. J., Reis, J. S. & Barbera-Stein, L. (1986). Family life education for young teens: An assessment of three interventions. *Health Education Quarterly*, **13**, 201–21.

140 REFERENCES

Heston, J. V. & Lazar, S. J. (1980). Evaluating a learning device for juvenile diabetics children. *Diabetes Care*, **3**, 688–71.

Hester, N. K. (1979). The pre-operational child's reaction to immunization. *Nursing Research*, **28**, 250–5.

Hilgard, J. K. & LeBaron, S. (1982). Relief of anxiety and pain in children and adolescents with cancer: Quantitative measures and clinical observations. *International Journal of Clinical and Experimental Hypnosis*, **30**, 417–22.

Hilgard, J. R. & Morgan, A. H. (1976). Treatment of anxiety and pain in childhood cancer through hypnosis. Paper presented to the 7th International Conference of Hypnosis and Psychosomatic Medicine, Philadelphia.

Hill, R. A., Britton, J. R. & Tattersfield, A. E. (1987). Management of asthma in schools. *Archives of Disease in Childhood*, **62**, 414–15.

Hill, R. A., Standen, P. J. & Tattersfield, A. E. (1989). Asthma, wheezing and school absence in primary schools. *Archives of Disease in Childhood*, **64**, 246–51.

Hirsch, B. (1980). Natural support systems and coping with major life changes. *American Journal of Community Psychology*, **8**, 263–77.

Hoare, P. (1987). Children with epilepsy and their families. *Journal of Child Psychology and Psychiatry*, **28**, 651–6.

Hobbs, N. & Perrin, J. M. (eds.) (1985). *Issues in the Care of Children with Chronic Illness.* San Francisco: Jossey Bass.

Holmes, H. A. & Holmes, F. F. (1975). After ten years, what are the handicaps and life-styles of children treated for cancer? An examination of the present status of 124 survivors. *Clinics in Pediatrics*, **14**, 819–23.

Hops, H. (1983). Children's social competence and skill: Current research practices and future directions. *Behavior Therapy*, **14**, 3–18.

Horowitz, M. J. & Kaltreider, N. B. (1980). Brief psychotherapy of stress response syndromes. In T. Karasu & L. Bellak (eds.), *Specialized Techniques in Individual Psychotherapy.* New York: Brunner/Mazel, pp. 162–83.

Hurtig, A. L., Koepke, D. & Park, K. B. (1989). Relation between severity of chronic illness and adjustment in children and adolescents with sickle cell disease. *Journal of Pediatric Psychology*, **14**, 117–32.

Hurtig, A. L. & White, L. S. (1986). Psychosocial adjustment in children and adolescents with sickle cell disease. *Journal of Pediatric Psychology*, **11**, 411–28.

Ingalls, A. & Salerno, M. (1971). *Maternal and Child Health Nursing.* St Louis: Mosby.

Ivey, J., Brewer, E. & Giannini, E. (1981). Psychosocial functioning in children with juvenile rheumatoid arthritis (JRA). *Arthritis and Rheumatology*, **24**, 5100.

Jay, S. M. & Elliott, C. H. (1984). Behavioral observation scales for measuring children's distress: The effects of increased methodological rigor. *Journal of Consulting and Clinical Psychology*, **52**, 1106–7.

Jay, S. M., Elliott, C., Katz, E. R. & Siegel, S. C. (1984). Stress reduction in children undergoing painful medical procedures. Paper presented at the Annual Meeting of the American Psychological Association, Toronto, Canada.

(1987). Cognitive-behavioral and pharmacologic interventions for children's distress during painful medical procedures. *Journal of Consulting and Clinical Psychology*, **55**, 860–5.

Jay, S. M., Elliott, C. H., Ozolins, M., Olson, R. & Pruitt, S. D. (1985). Behavioral management of children's distress during painful medical procedures. *Behavior Research and Therapy*, **23**, 513–20.

Johnson, S. B. (1988). Psychological aspects of childhood diabetes. *Journal of Child Psychology and Psychiatry*, **29**, 729–39.

Johnson, S. B., Pollak, T., Silverstein, J. H., Rosenbloom, A. L., Spiller, R., McCallum, M. & Harkavy, J. (1982). Cognitive and behavioral knowledge about insulin dependent diabetes among children and parents. *Pediatrics*, **69**, 708–13.

Johnston, C. C. & Strada, M. E. (1986). Acute pain response in infants: a multidimensional description. *Pain*, **24**, 373–82.

Jones, R. T., Kazdin, A. E. & Haney, J. I. (1981). Social validation and training of emergency fire safety skills for potential injury prevention and life-saving. *Journal of Applied Behavior Analysis*, **14**, 249–60.

Kagan, J. (1983). Stress and coping in early development. In N. Garmezy & M. Rutter (eds.), *Stress, Coping, and Development in Children*. New York: McGraw-Hill, pp. 191–216.

Kagen, L. B. (1976). Use of denial in adolescents with bone cancer. *Health and Social Work*, **1**, 71–87.

Kaplan, R. M., Chadwick, M. W. & Schimmel, L. E. (1985). Social learning intervention to promote metabolic control in type 1 diabetes mellitus: Pilot experiment results. *Diabetes Care*, **8**, 152–5.

Kaplan, D. M., Grobstein, R. & Smith, A. (1976). Predicting the impact of severe illness in families. *Health and Social Work*, **1**, 71–82.

Kaplan, D. M., Smith, A., Grobstein, R. & Fischman, S. E. (1973). Family mediation of stress. *Social Work*, **18**, 60–9.

Karoly, P. (1982). Developmental paediatrics: A process-oriented approach to the analysis of health competence. In P. Karoly, J. J. Steffen & D. J. O'Grady (eds.), *Child Health Psychology: Concepts and Issues*. New York: Pergamon Press, pp. 29–57.

Kashani, J. H., Koenig, P., Shepperd, J. A., Wilfley, D. & Morris, D. A. (1988). Psychopathology and self-concept in asthmatic children. *Journal of Pediatric Psychology*, **13**, 509–20.

Kastenbaum, R. & Costa, P. T. Jnr. (1977). Psychological perspectives on death. *Annual Review of Psychology*, **28**, 225–49.

Katz, E. R., Kellerman, J., Rigler, D., Williams, K. O. & Siegel, S. E.

(1977). School intervention with pediatric cancer patients. *Journal of Pediatric Psychology*, **2**, 72–6.

Katz, E. R., Kellerman, J. & Siegel, S. E. (1980). Distress behavior in children with cancer undergoing medical procedures: Developmental considerations. *Journal of Consulting and Clinical Psychology*, **48**, 356–65.

Kazak, A. E. & Clark, M. W. (1986). Stress in families of children with myelaneningocele. *Developmental Medicine and Child Neurology*, **28**, 220–8.

Kazak, A. E., Reber, M. & Carter, A. (1988). Structural and qualitative aspects of social networks in families with young chronically ill children. *Journal of Pediatric Psychology*, **13**, 171–82.

Kazak, A. & Wilcox, B. (1984). The structure and function of social support networks in families with a handicapped child. *American Journal of Community Psychology*, **12**, 645–61.

Kazdin, A. E. (1989). Developmental psychopathology: Current research, issues and directions. *American Psychologist*, **44**, 180–7.

Kendrick, C., Culling, J., Oakhill, T. & Mott, M. (1986). Children's understanding of their illness and its treatment within a paediatric oncology unit. *Association for Child Psychology and Psychiatry* (Newsletter), **8**, 16–20.

Keneally, T. (1978). *Ned Kelly and the City of the Bees*. England: Puffin Books.

King, E. H. (1981). Child-rearing practices: Child with chronic illness and well sibling. *Issues in Comprehensive Pediatric Nursing*, **5**, 105–94.

Klinzing, D. R. & Klinzing, D. G. (1977). Communicating with young children about hospitalization. *Communication Education*, **26**, 307–13.

Koocher, G. P. (1973). Childhood, death and cognitive development. *Developmental Psychology*, **9**, 369–75.

(1980). Initial consultations with the pediatric cancer patient. In J. Kellerman (ed.), *Psychological Aspects of Childhood Cancer*. New York: Charles Thomas.

(1981). Children's conceptions of death. In R. Bibace & M. E. Walsh (eds.), *Children's Conceptions of Health, Illness and Bodily Functions*. San Francisco: Jossey Bass, pp. 85–100.

Koocher, G. P. & O'Malley, J. E. (1981). Implications for patient care. In G. P. Koocher & J. E. O'Malley (eds.), *The Damodes Syndrome: Psychosocial Consequences of Surviving Childhood Cancer*. New York: McGraw-Hill.

Korsch, B. M., Fine, R. & Negrette, V. G. (1978). Noncompliance in children with renal transplants. *Pediatrics*, **61**, 872–6.

Kovacs, M. (1981). Rating scales to assess depression in school-aged children. *Acta Paedopsychiatrica*, **46**, 305–15.

Kovacs, M., Feinberg, T. L., Paulauskas, S., Finkelstein, R., Pollock, M. & Crouse-Novak, M. (1985). Initial coping responses and psychosocial characteristics of children with insulin-dependent diabetes mellitus. *Journal of Pediatrics*, **106**, 827–42.

Kubany, A. J., Danowski, T. S. & Moses, C. (1956). The personality and intelligence of diabetics. *Diabetes*, **5**, 462–7.

Kubler-Ross, E. (1969). *On Death and Dying*. New York: Macmillan.

Kupst, M. J. & Schulman, J. L. (1988). Long-term coping with pediatric leukemia: A six-year follow-up study. *Journal of Pediatric Psychology*, **13**, 7–22.

Kupst, M. J., Schulman, J. L., Honig, G., Maurer, H., Morgan, E. & Fochtman, D. (1982). Family coping with childhood leukemia: One year after diagnosis. *Journal of Pediatric Psychology*, **7**, 157–74.

Kupst, M. J., Schulman, J. L., Maurer, H., Morgan, E., Honig, G. & Fochtman, D. (1984). Coping with pediatric leukemia: A two-year follow-up. *Journal of Pediatric Psychology*, **9**, 149–63.

Kuttner, L. (1984). Psychological treatment of distress, pain, and anxiety for young children with cancer. Unpublished doctoral dissertation, Simon Frazer University.

La Greca, A. M. (1982). Behavioral aspects of diabetes management in children and adolescents. *Diabetes*, **31** (Suppl.), 47 (Abstract).

(1988). Adherence to prescribed medical regimens. In D. Routh (ed.), *Handbook of Pediatric Psychology*. New York: Guilford Press, pp. 299 –320.

Lacey, J. I. (1967). Somatic response patterning and stress. In M. H. Appley & R. Trumball (eds.), *Psychological Stress: Issues in Research*. New York: Appley-Century-Crofts.

Lamb, M. E. & Sutton-Smith, D. (eds.) (1982). *Sibling Relationships: Their Nature and Significance across the Life-span*. Hillsdale, NJ: Erlbaum.

Lancaster, S., Prior, M. & Adler, R. (1989). Child behavior ratings: the influence of maternal characteristics and child temperament. *Journal of Child Psychology and Psychiatry*, **30**, 137–50.

Lansky, S., Cairns, N., Hassanein, R., Wehr, J. & Lowman, J. T. (1978). Childhood cancer: Parental discord and divorce. *Pediatrics*, **62**, 184–8.

Lansky, S. B., Cairns, N. & Zwartjes, W. (1983). School attendance among children with cancer: A report from two centres. *Journal of Psychosocial Oncology*, **1**, 75–82.

Lansky, S. B., Lowman, J. T., Vats, T. & Gyulay, J.-E. (1975). School phobia in children with malignant neoplasms. *American Journal of Diseases of Children*, **129**, 42–6.

Laurence, K. M. & Tew, B. J. (1971). Natural history of spina bifida cystica and cranium bifidum cysticum: Major central nervous system malformations in South Wales, Part IV. *Archives of Disease in Childhood*, **46**, 127–38.

Lavigne, J. V. & Burns, W. J. (1981). *Pediatric Psychology: Introduction for Pediatricians and Psychologists*. New York: Grune & Stratton.

Lazarus, R. S. (1966). *Psychological Stress and the Coping Process*. New York: McGraw-Hill.

Lazarus, R. S. & Folkman, S. (1984). *Stress, Appraisal and Coping*. New York: Springer.

LeBaron, S. & Hilgard, J. (1984). *Hypnotherapy of Pain in Children with Cancer*. Los Alton, CA: William Kaufman.

Leiderman, P. H. (1983). Social ecology and childbirth: The newborn nursery as environmental stress. In N. Garmezy & M. Rutter (eds.), *Stress, Coping and Development in Children*. New York: McGraw-Hill, pp. 133–59.

Lemanek, K. L., Moore, S. L., Gresham, F. M., Williamson, D. A. & Kelley, M. L. (1986). Psychological adjustment of children with sickle cell anemia. *Journal of Pediatric Psychology*, **11**, 397–426.

Levenson, P. M., Copeland, D. R., Morrow, J. R., Pfefferbaum, B. & Silberberg, Y. (1983). Disparities in disease-related perceptions of adolescent cancer patients and their parents. *Journal of Pediatric Psychology*, **8**, 33–45.

Leventhal, H. (1982). The integration of emotion and cognition: A view from the perceptual motor theory of emotion. In M. S. Clarke & S. T. Fiske (eds.), *Affect and Cognition: The Seventeenth Annual Carnegie Symposium on Cognition*. Hillsdale, NJ: Lawrence Erlbaum Ass., Inc.

Levin, I. (1986). *Stage and Structure*. New Jersey: Ablex.

Lewis, C. & Lewis, M. (1982). Determinants of children's health related beliefs and behaviors. *Family and Community Health*, **2**, 85–97.

Lewis, C. E., Rachelsefsky, G., Lewis, M. A., de la Suta, A. & Kaplan, M. (1984). A randomized trial of A.C.T. (Asthma Care Training) for kids. *Pediatrics*, **74**, 478–86.

Ley, P. (1982). Giving information to patients. In J. R. Eiser (ed.), *Social Psychology and Behavioral Medicine*. New York: Wiley.

Lindemann, J. E. (ed.) (1981). *Psychological and Behavioral Aspects of Physical Disabilaity*. New York: Plenum Press.

Lineberger, H. O. (1981). Social characteristics of a hemophilia clinic population. *General Hospital Psychiatry*, **3**, 157–63.

Linn, S. (1978). Puppet therapy in hospitals: Helping children cope. *Journal of the American Medical Women's Association*, **33**, 61–5.

Linn, S., Beardslee, W. & Patenaude, A. F. (1986). Puppet therapy with pediatric Bone Marrow Transplant Patients. *Journal of Pediatric Psychology*, **11**, 37–46.

Lipowski, Z. J. (1971). Physical illness, the individual and the coping process. *Psychiatry in Medicine*, **1**, 91–8.

Lipsitt, L. P. (1958). A self-concept scale for children and its relation to the children's form of manifest anxiety. *Child Development*, **29**, 463–72.

Litt, I., Cuskey, W. & Rosenberg, A. (1982). Role of self-esteem and autonomy in determining medication compliance among adolescents with juvenile rheumatoid arthritis. *Pediatrics*, **69**, 15.

Lobato, D., Barbour, L., Hall, L. J. & Miller, C. T. (1987). Psychosocial characteristics of preschool siblings of handicapped and non-handicapped children. *Journal of Abnormal Child Psychology*, **15**, 329–38.

Lobato, D., Faust, D & Spirito, A. (1988). Examining the effects of chronic disease and disability on children's sibling relationships. *Journal of Pediatric Psychology*, **13**, 389–408.

Lorenz, R., Christensen, N. & Pichert, J. (1985). Diet-related knowledge, skilled adherence among children with insulin-dependent diabetes mellitus. *Pediatrics*, **75**.

Maccoby, E. E. (1984). Middle childhood in the context of the family. In W. A. Collins (ed.), *Development during Middle Childhood*. Washington, DC: The Academy Press, pp. 184–239.

Madden, N. A., Terrizzi, J. & Friedman, S. B. (1982). Psychological issues in mothers of children with hemophilia. *Journal of Developmental and Behavioral Pediatrics*, **3**, 136–42.

Maddux, J. E., Roberts, M. C., Sleddon, E. A. & Wright, L. (1986). Developmental issues in child health psychology. *American Psychologist*, **41**, 25–34.

Malone, J., Hellrung, I., Malphus, E., Rosenbloom, A. L., Grgic, M. D. & Weber, F. T. (1976). Good diabetic control: A study in mass delusion. *Journal of Pediatrics*, **88**, 943–7.

Malpas, J. S. (1988). Cancer: The consequences of cure. *Clinical Radiology*, **39**, 166–72.

Mandler, J. (1983). Representation. In J. H. Flavell & E. H. Markman (eds.), *Handbook of Child Psychology*, Vol. III: *Cognitive Development*. New York: Wiley.

Markova, I., MacDonald, K. & Forbes, C. (1980). Integration of haemophilic boys into normal schools. *Child: Care, Health and Development*, **6**, 101–9.

Marteau, T. M., Bloch, S. & Baum, J. D. (1987). Family life and diabetic control. *Journal of Child Psychology and Psychiatry*, **28**, 823–34.

Martin, A. J., Landau, L. I. & Phelan, P. D. (1982). Asthma from childhood at age 21: The patient and his disease. *British Medical Journal*, **284**, 380–2.

Mattson, A. & Agle, D. P. (1972). Group therapy with parents of hemophiliacs: Therapeutic process and observations of parental adaptation to chronic illness in children. *Journal of the American Academy of Child Psychiatry*, **11**, 558–71.

McAlister, R., Butler, E. & Lei, T. (1973). Patterns of interaction among families of behaviorally retarded children. *Journal of Marriage and the Family*, **35**, 93–100.

McAnarney, E. R., Pless, I. B., Satterwhite, B. & Friedman, S. (1974). Psychological problems of children with chronic juvenile arthritis. *Pediatrics*, **53**, 523.

McAndrew, I. (1979). Adolescents and young people with spina bifida. *Developmental Medicine and Child Neurology*, **21**, 619–29.

McCrae, R. R. & Costa, P. T. Jnr. (1986). Personality, coping and coping effectiveness in an adult sample. *Journal of Personality*, **54**, 919–28.

McDonald, A. C., Carson, K. L., Palmer, D. J. & Slay, T. (1982).

Physicians' diagnostic information to parents of handicapped neonates. *Mental Retardation*, **20**, 12–14.

McFadden, E. R. Jr. (1980). Asthma: Pathophysiology. *Seminars in Respiratory Medicine*, **1**, 297–303.

McGarvey, M. E. (1983). Preschool hospital tours. *Children's Health Care*, **11**, 122–4.

McGrath, P. J., Johnson, G., Goodman, J. R., Schillinger, J., Dunn, J. & Chapman, J. (1985). The CHEOPS: A behavioral scale to measure post operative pain in children. In H. L. Fields, R. Dubner & F. Cervero (eds.), *Advances in Pain Research and Therapy*. New York: Raven Press, pp. 395–402.

McGrath, P. J. & Unruh, A. M. (1987). *Pain in Children and Adolescents*. Amsterdam: Elsevier.

McHale, S. & Gamble, W. (1987). Relationship between handicapped children and their non-handicapped siblings and peers. In J. Garbarino, T. Brookhauser & K. Authier (eds.), *Special Children – Special Risks: The Maltreatment of Handicapped Children*. New York: Aldine.

McHale, S. M. & Simeonsson, R. J. (1980). Effects of interactions on non-handicapped children's attitudes toward autistic children. *American Journal of Mental Deficiency*, **85**, 18–24.

McNabb, W. L., Wilson-Pessano, S. R. & Jacobs, A. M. (1986). Critical self-management competencies for children with asthma. *Journal of Pediatric Psychology*, **11**, 103–18.

Mearig, J. S. (1985). Cognitive development of chronically ill children. In N. Hobbs & J. M. Perrin (eds.), *Issues in the Care of Children with Chronic Illness*. San Francisco: Jossey Bass.

Mechanic, D. (1980). The experience and reporting of common symptoms. *Journal of Health and Social Behavior*, **21**, 146–55.

(1983). The experience and expression of distress: The study of illness behavior and medical utilization. In D. Mechanic (ed.), *The Challenge of Pain*. Harmondsworth: Penguin, pp. 195–261.

Mechanic, D. & Hansell, S. (1987). Adolescent competence, psychological well-being and self-assessed physical health. *Journal of Health and Social Behavior*, **28**, 364–74.

Meichenbaum, D. (1975). Self-instructional methods. In F. H. Kaufer & A. P. Goldstein (eds.), *Helping People Change*. New York: Pergamon Press, pp. 357–92.

Meijer, A. (1980). Psychiatric problems of hemophilic boys and their families. *International Journal of Psychiatry in Medicine*, **10**, 163–72.

Melamed, B. G. (1981). Effects of preparatory information on the adjustment of children to medical procedures. In M. Rosenbaum & C. M. Franks (eds.), *Perspectives on Behavior Therapy in the Eighties*. New York: Springer Verlag.

Meltzer, J., Bibace, R. & Walsh, M. E. (1984). Children's conceptions of smoking. *Journal of Pediatric Psychology*, **9**, 41–56.

Melzack, R. (1975). The McGill pain questionnaire: Major properties and scoring methods. *Pain*, 1, 277–99.

Melzack, R. (ed.) (1983). *Pain Measurement and Assessment*. New York: Raven Press, pp. 1–6.

Merskey, H. (ed.) (1986). Classification of chronic pain: descriptions of chronic pain syndromes and definitions of pain terms. *Pain*, suppl. 3.

Michela, J. L. & Contento, I. R. (1984). Spontaneous classification of foods by elementary school-aged children. *Health Education Quarterly*, 11, 57–76.

Miller, J., Spitz, P., Simpson, U. & Williams, G. (1982). The social function of young adults who had arthritis in childhood. *Pediatrics*, 100, 378.

Miller, S. (1987). Monitoring and blunting: Validation of a questionnaire to assess styles of information seeking under threat. *Journal of Personality and Social Psychology*, 52, 345–53.

Minuchin, S., Baker, L., Rosman, B., Leibman, R., Milman, L. & Todd, T. (1975). A conceptual model of psychosomatic illness in children. *Archives of General Psychiatry*, 32, 1031–8.

Mitchell, R. & Trickett, E. (1980). Social networks and mediators of social support: An analysis of the effects and determinants of social networks. *Community Mental Health Journal*, 16, 27–44.

Moos, R. G. & Moos, B. S. (1981). *Family Environment Scale*. Palo Alto, CA: Consulting Psychologists Press.

Morgan, S. A. & Jackson, J. (1986). Psychological and social concomitants of sickle cell anemia. *Journal of Pediatric Psychology*, 11, 429–40.

Morrow, G. R., Carpenter, P. J. & Hoagland, A. C. (1984). The role of social support in parental adjustment to pediatric cancer. *Journal of Pediatric Psychology*, 9, 317–30.

Mrazek, D. A. (1986). Childhood asthma: two central questions for child psychiatry. *Journal of Child Psychology and Psychiatry*, 27, 1–6.

Mrazek, D., Anderson, I. & Strunk, R. (1985). Disturbed emotional development of severely asthmatic pre-school children. In J. E. Stevenson (ed.), *Recent Research in Developmental Psychopathology*. Oxford: Pergamon, pp. 81–93.

Mulhern, R. K., Crisco, J. J. & Camitta, B. M. (1981). Patterns of communication among pediatric patients with leukemia, parents, and physicians: Prognostic disagreements and misunderstandings. *Journal of Pediatrics*, 99, 480–3.

Mulhern, R. K., Ochs, J., Fairclough, D. (1987). Intellectual and academic achievement status after CNS relapse: A retrospective study of 40 children treated for acute lymphoblastic leukemia. *Journal of Clinical Oncology*, 5, 933–40.

Mulhern, R. K., Wasserman, A. L., Friedman, A. G. & Fairclough, D. (1989). Social competence and behavioral adjustment of children who are long-term survivors of cancer. *Pediatrics*, 83, 18–25.

Myers, B. A. (1983). The informing interview. *American Journal of Diseases of Children*, **137**, 572–7.

Myers-Vando, R., Steward, M. S., Folkins, C. H. & Hynes, P. (1979). The effects of congenital heart disease on cognitive development, illness causality concepts, and vulnerability. *American Journal of Ortho-psychiatry*, **49**, 617–24.

Natapoff, J. (1978). Children's views of health. *American Journal of Public Health*, **68**, 995–1000.

Nelson, K. (ed.) (1986). *Event Knowledge: Structure and Function in Development*. New Jersey: Lawrence Erlbaum.

Nelson, K. & Gruendel, J. (1986). Children's scripts. In K. Nelson (ed.), *Event Knowledge: Structure and Function in Development*. New Jersey: Lawrence Erlbaum.

Nimorwicz, P. & Klein, R. H. (1986). Psychosocial aspects of hemophilia in families: II. Intervention strategies and procedures. *Clinical Psychology Review*, **2**, 171–81.

Nolan, T., Desmond, K., Herlich, R. & Hardy, S. (1986). Knowledge of cystic fibrosis in patients and their parents. *Pediatrics*, **77**, 229–35.

Norrish, M., Tooley, M. & Godfrey, S. (1977). Clinical, physiological, and psychological study of asthmatic children attending a hospital clinic. *Archives of Disease in Childhood*, **52**, 912–17.

Novak, D., Plummer, R. & Smith, R. (1979). Changes in physicians' attitudes toward telling the cancer patient. *Journal of the American Medical Association*, **241**, 897–900.

Nowicki, S. & Strickland, B. R. (1973). A locus of control scale for children. *Journal of Consulting and Clinical Psychology*, **40**, 148–54.

Obetz, S. W., Swenson, W. M., McCarthy, C. A., Gilchrist, G. S. & Burgert, E. O. (1980). Children who survive malignant disease: Emotional adaptation of the children and their families. In J. L. Schulman & M. J. Kupst (eds.), *The Child with Cancer: Clinical Approaches to Psychosocial Care – Research in Psychosocial Aspects*. Springfield, IL: Charles C. Thomas, pp. 194–210.

Olch, D. (1971). Effects of hemophilia upon intellectual growth and academic achievement. *Journal of Genetic Psychology*, **119**, 63–74.

Olness, K. (1981). Imagery (self-hypnosis) as adjunct therapy in childhood cancer. *American Journal of Pediatric Hematology-Oncology*, **3**, 313–21.

Orr, D. P., Weller, S. C., Satterwhite, B. & Pless, I. B. (1984). Psychosocial implications of chronic illness in adolescence. *Journal of Pediatrics*, **194**, 152–7.

Pantell, R. H., Stewart, T. J., Dias, J. K., Wells, P. & Ross, A. W. (1982). Physician communication with children and parents. *Pediatrics*, **70**, 396–402.

Parcel, G. S., Nader, P. R. & Tiernan, D. (1980). Impact of a health education programme for children with asthma. Paper presented at the Ambulatory Pediatric Association Meeting, San Antonio.

Parker, J. G. & Asher, S. R. (1987). Peer relations and later adjustment: Are low-accepted children 'at risk'? *Psychological Bulletin*, **102**, 357–89.

Peckham, V. C., Meadows, A. T., Bartel, N. & Marrero, O. (1988). Educational late effects in long-term survivors of childhood acute lymphocytic leukemia. *Pediatrics*, **81**, 127–33.

Pennebaker, J. W., Cox, D. J., Gonder-Frederick, L., Wunsch, M. G., Evans, W. S. & Pohl, S. (1981). Physical symptoms related to blood glucose in insulin-dependent diabetes. *Psychosomatic Medicine*, **43**, 489–500.

Pentz, M. A. (1980). Assertion training and trainer effects on unassertive and aggressive adolescents. *Journal of Counselling Psychology*, **27**, 76–83.

Perrin, E. C. & Gerrity, P. S. (1981). There's a demon in your belly: Children's understanding of illness. *Pediatrics*, **67**, 841–9.

(1984). Development of children with a chronic illness. *Pediatric Clinics of North America*, **31**, 19–31.

Perrin, E. C., Ramsey, B. K. & Sandler, H. M. (1987). Competent kids: Children and adolescents with a chronic illness. *Child Care, Health and Development*, **13**, 13–32.

Perrin, J. M. & MacLean, W. E. (1987). *Education and Stress Management in Childhood Chronic Illness*. Final report to William T. Grant Foundation, Grant No. 82-0836-00.

Perrin, J. M., MacLean, W. E. & Perrin, E. C. (1989). Parental perceptions of health status and psychologic adjustment of children with asthma. *Pediatrics*, **83**, 26–30.

Perrin, J. M. & MacLean, W. E. Jr. (1988). Children with chronic illness: The prevention of dysfunction. *Pediatric Clinics of North America*, **35**, 1325–37.

Peshkin, M. M. (1930). Asthma in children: IX. Role of environment in the treatment of a selected group of cases: A plea for a 'home' as a restorative environment. *American Journal of Diseases of Children*, **39**, 774–81.

Peterson, C. & Brownlee-Duffeck, M. (1984). Prevention of anxiety and pain due to medical and dental procedures. In M. C. Roberts & L. Peterson (eds.), *Prevention of Problems in Childhood: Psychological Research and Applications*. New York: Wiley.

Peterson, L. & Mori, L. (1988). Preparation for hospitalization. In D. Routh (ed.), *Handbook of Pediatric Psychology*. New York: Guilford Press, pp. 460–91.

Peterson, L. & Ridley-Johnson, R. (1980). Pediatric hospital response to survey of prehospital preparation for children. *Journal of Pediatric Psychology*, **5**, 1–7.

(1983). Prevention of disorders in children. In C. E. Walker & M. C. Roberts (eds.), *Handbook of Clinical Child Psychology*. New York: Wiley.

Peterson, L., Schultheis, K., Ridley-Johnson, R., Miller, D. J. & Tracy, K.

(1984). Comparison of three modeling procedures on the presurgical and postsurgical reactions of children. *Behavior Therapy*, **15**, 197–203.

Peterson, L. & Shigetomi, C. (1981). The use of coping techniques to minimize anxiety in hospitalized children. *Behavior Therapy*, **12**, 1–14.

(1982). One-year follow-up of behavioral presurgical preparation for children. *Journal of Pediatric Psychology*, **7**, 43–8.

(1983). One-year follow-up of elective surgery child patients receiving preoperative preparation. *Journal of Pediatric Psychology*, **7** (1), 43–8.

Piaget, J. (1929). *The Child's Conception of the World*. New York: Harcourt Brace.

Piaget, J. & Inhelder, B. (1969). *The Psychology of the Child*. New York: Basic Books.

Piers, E. Y. (1969). *Manual for the Piera-Harris Children's Self-concept Scale (The way I feel about myself)*. Nashville, TN: Counselor Researchings and Tests.

Pinto, R. P. & Hollandsworth, J. G. Jnr. (1984). Preparing parents of pediatric surgical patients using a videotape model. Paper presented at the meeting of the Society of Behavioral Medicine, Philadelphia.

Plank, E. (1964). Death on a Children's Ward. *Medical Times*, **92**, 638–44.

Platt Committee, Great Britain (1959). *The Welfare of Children in Hospitals*. London: Her Majesty's Stationery Office.

Pless, I. B. & Pinkerton, P. (1975). *Chronic Childhood Disorder: Promoting Patterns of Adjustment*. London: Henry Kimpton.

Pless, I. B. & Roghmann, K. J. (1971). Chronic illness and its consequences: Observations based on three epidemiological surveys. *Journal of Pediatrics*, **79**, 351–9.

Porter, C. (1974). Grade school children's perceptions of their internal body parts. *Nursing Research*, **23**, 384–91.

Potter, P. C. & Roberts, M. C. (1984). Children's perceptions of chronic illness: The roles of disease symptoms, cognitive development and information. *Journal of Pediatric Psychology*, **9**, 13–28.

Powell, T. H. & Ogle, P. A. (1985). *Brothers and Sisters – A Special Part of Exceptional Families*. Baltimore: Paul H. Brookes.

Quinton, D. & Rutter, M. (1976). Early hospital admissions and later disturbances of behavior: An attempted replication of Douglas findings. *Developmental Medicine and Child Neurology*, **18**, 447–59.

Rachman, S. & Phillips, C. (1975). *Psychology and Medicine*. London: Temple Smith.

Rando, T. A. (1983). An investigation of grief and adaptation in parents whose children have died from cancer. *Journal of Pediatric Psychology*, **8**, 3–20.

Rapoff, M. A. & Christophersen, E. R. (1982). Improving compliance in pediatric practice. *Pediatric Clinics of North America*, **29**, 339–57.

Rawls, D. J., Rawls, J. R. & Harrison, C. W. (1971). An investigation of six-to eleven-year-old children with allergic disorders. *Journal of Consulting and Clinical Psychology*, **36**, 260–4.

Redpath, C. C. & Rogers, C. S. (1984). Healthy young children's concepts of hospitals, medical personnel, operations and illness. *Journal of Pediatric Psychology*, **9**, 29–40.

Reilly, T. P., Hasazi, J. E. & Bond, L. A. (1983). Children's conceptions of death and personal mortality. *Journal of Pediatric Psychology*, **8**, 21–32.

Reiss, D. (1982). *The Family's Construction of Reality*. Cambridge, MA: Harvard University Press.

Renne, C. M. & Creer, T. L. (1985). Asthmatic children and their families. *Advances in Developmental and Behavioral Pediatrics* (Vol. 6). Greenwich, CT: JAI Press.

Richardson, G. M., McGrath, P. J., Cunningham, S. J. & Humphreys, P. (1983). Validity of the headache diary for children. *Headache*, **23**, 184–7.

Roberts, M. & Peterson, L. (eds.) (1984). *Prevention of Problems in Childhood*. New York: Wiley.

Roberts, M. C., Wortele, S. K., Boone, R. R., Ginther, L. J. & Elkins. P. D. (1981). Reduction of medical fears by use of modeling: A preventive application in a general population of children. *Journal of Pediatric Psychology*, **6**, 293–300.

Robertson, J. (1952). *A two-year-old goes to hospital* [Film]. New York: New York University Film Library.

Robertson, J. (1958). *Young Children in Hospitals*. New York: Basic Books.

Rodin, J. (1983). *Will This Hurt?* London: Royal College of Nursing.

Rosch, E. (1978). Principles of categorization. In E. Rosch & B. B. Lloyd (eds.), *Cognition and Categorization*. Hillsdale, NJ: L. Erlbaum.

Rosenbaum, P. L., Armstrong, R. W. & King, S. M. (1986). Children's attitudes toward disabled peers: a self-report measure. *Journal of Pediatric Psychology*, **11**, 517–30.

Roskies, E., Mongeon, M. & Gagnon-Lefebvre, B. (1978). Increasing maternal participation in the hospitalization of young children. *Medical Care*, **16**, 765–77.

Ross, D. M. & Ross, S. A. (1984a). Childhood pain: the school-aged child's viewpoint. *Pain*, **20**, 179–91.

(1984b). Teaching the child with leukemia to cope with teasing. *Issues in Comprehensive Pediatric Nursing*, **7**, 59–66.

Rovet, J. F., Ehrlich, R. M. & Hoppe, M. (1987). Intellectual deficits associated with early onset of insulin-dependent diabetes mellitus in children. *Diabetes Care*, **10**, 510–15.

Rubin, D. H., Leventhal, J. M., Sadock, R. T., Letovsky, E., Schottland, P., Clemente, I. & McCarthy, P. (1986). Educational intervention by computer in childhood asthma: A randomized clinical trial testing the use of a new teaching intervention in childhood asthma. *Pediatrics*, **77**, 1–10.

Rutter, M. (1981). Stress, coping and development: Some issues and some questions. *Journal of Child Psychology and Psychiatry*, **22**, 323–56.

Rutter, M., Graham, P. & Yule, W. (1970). *Clinics in Developmental Medicine*: No. 35/36 *A Neuropsychiatric Study in Childhood*. London: SIMP/Heinemann.

Rutter, M., Tizard, J. & Whitmore, K. (1970). *Education, Health, and Behaviour*. London: Longman Press.

Ryan, C., Vega, A. & Drash, A. (1985). Cognitive deficits in adolescents who developed diabetes early in life. *Pediatrics*, **75**, 921–7.

Sabbeth, B. F. & Leventhal, J. M. (1984). Marital adjustment to chronic childhood illness: A critique of the literature. *Pediatrics*, **73**, 762–8.

Saille, H., Burgmeier, R. & Schmidt, L. R. (1988). A meta-analysis of studies on psychological preparation of children facing medical procedures *Psychology and Health*, **2**, 107–32.

Saunders, A. M. & Lamb, W. (1977). A group experience with parents of hemophilics: A viable alternative to group therapy. *Journal of Clinical Child Psychology*, **6**, 79–82.

Savedra, M., Gibbons, P., Tesler, M., Ward, J. & Wegner, C. (1982). How do children describe pain? A tentative assessment. *Pain*, **14**, 95–104.

Scamagas, P. & Rodabaugh, B. (1981). Development and evaluation of a self-management system for children with asthma. In *Self-Management Educational Programme for Childhood Asthma*. Bethesda, MD: National Institute of Allergy and Infectious Diseases, Vol. 2, pp. 129–50.

Schechter, N. L., Allen, D. A. & Hanson, K. (1986). Status of pediatric pain control: A comparison of hospital analgesic usage in children and adults. *Pediatrics*, **77**, 11–15.

Schilder, P. & Wechsler, D. (1935). What do children know about the interior of the body? *International Journal of Psychoanalysis*, **16**, 345–50.

Schinke, S. P. (1981). Interpersonal skills training with adolescents. In M. Hersen, R. M. Eisler & P. M. Miller (eds.), *Progress in Behavior Modification*, Vol. II. New York: Academic Press.

Schwirian, P. M. (1976). Effects of the presence of a hearing-impaired preschool child in the family on behavior patterns of older 'normal' siblings. *American Annals of the Deaf*, **121**, 373–80.

Selman, R. L. (1980). *The Growth of Interpersonal Understanding*. New York: Academic Press.

Sergis-Deavenport, E. & Varni, J. W. (1982). Behavioral techniques in teaching hemophilia factor replacement procedures to families. *Pediatric Nursing*, **8**, 416–19.

(1983). Behavioral assessment of adherence to factor replacement therapy in hemophilia. *Journal of Pediatric Psychology*, **8**, 367–77.

Shannon, F. T., Ferguson, D. M. & Dimond, M. E. (1984). Early hospital admissions and subsequent behavior problems in 6-year-olds. *Archives of Disease in Childhood*, **59**, 815–19.

Shapiro, E. K. & Wallace, D. B. (1987). Siblings and parents in one-parent families. *Journal of Children in Contemporary Society*, **19**, 91–114.

Share, L. (1972). Family communication in the crisis of a child's fatal illness: A literature review and analysis. *Omega*, **3** (3), 187–201.

Shipp, J. C. (1963). Florida's first summer camp for diabetic children. *Journal of the Florida Medical Association*, **50**, 133.

Shope, J. T. (1981). Medication compliance. *Pediatric Clinics of North America*, **28**, 5–21.

Siegel, S. C., Katz, R. M. & Rachelefsky, G. S. (1983). Asthma in infancy and childhood. In E. Middleton, Jnr., C. E. Reed & E. F. Ellis (eds.), *Allergy: Principles and Practice* (2nd edn), St Louis: Mosby.

Silver, R. L. & Wortman, C. B. (1980). Coping with undesirable life events. In J. Garber & M. E. P. Seligman (eds.), *Human Helplessness: Theory and Applications*. New York: Academic Press, pp. 279–340.

Silverstein, J. H., Rosenbloom, A. L., Clarke, D. W., Spillar, R. & Pendergast, J. F. (1983). Accuracy of two systems for blood glucose monitoring without a meter (Chemstrip/Visidex). *Diabetes Care*, **6**, 533–5.

Simonds, J. F. (1979). Emotions and compliance in diabetic children. *Psychosomatics*, **20**, 544–51.

Skipper, J. K. Jnr., Leonard, R. L. & Rhymes, J. (1968). Child hospitalization and social interaction: An experimental study of mothers' feelings of stress, adaptation and satisfaction. *Medical Care*, **6**, 496–506.

Slavin, L. A., O'Malley, J. E., Koocher, G. & Foster, D. J. (1982). Communication of the cancer diagnosis to pediatric patients: Impact on long-term adjustment. *American Journal of Psychiatry*, **139** (2), 179–83.

Soissignan, R., Koch, P. & Montagner, H. (1988). Behavioral and cardiovascular changes in children moving from Kindergarten to primary school. *Journal of Child Psychology and Psychiatry*, **29**, 321–34.

Sourkes, B. (1977). Facilitating family coping with childhood cancer. *Journal of Pediatric Psychology*, **2**, 65–7.

Spaulding, B. R. & Morgan, S. B. (1986). Spina bifida children and their parents: A population prone to family dysfunction. *Journal of Pediatric Psychology*, **11**, 359–74.

Spencer, R. F. (1971). Psychiatric impairment versus adjustment in hemophilia: Review and five case studies. *Psychiatry in Medicine*, **2**, 1–12.

Spinetta, J. J. (1980). Disease-related communication: How to tell. In J. Kellerman (ed.), *Psychological Aspects of Childhood Cancer*. Springfield, IL: Thomas.

(1981). Adjustment and adaptation in children with cancer. In J. J. Spinetta & P. Spinetta (eds.), *Living with Childhood Cancer*. St Louis: Mosby.

(1982). Psychosocial issues in childhood cancer: How the professional can help. In M. Wolraich & D. K. Routh (eds.), *Advances in Developmental and Behavioral Pediatrics* (Vol. 3). Greenwich, CT: JAI Press.

Spinetta, J., Rigler, D. & Karon, M. (1973). Anxiety in the dying child. *Pediatrics*, **52**, 841–5.

Spinetta, J. J. & Spinetta, P. (eds.) (1981). *Living with Childhood Cancer*. St Louis: C. V. Mosby.

Spinetta, J. J., Swarner, J. A. & Sheposh, J. P. (1981). Effective parental coping following the death of a child from cancer. *Journal of Pediatric Psychology*, **6**, 251–63.

Spinetta, P. & Spinetta, J. J. (1980). The child with cancer in school: Teacher's appraisal. *American Journal of Pediatric Hematology/Ongology*, **2**, 89–94.

Spirito, A., Stark, L. J. & Tye, V. (1989). Common coping strategies employed by children with chronic illness. *Newsletter of the Society of Pediatric Psychology*, **13**, 3–8.

Spirito, A., Stark, L. J. & Williams, C. (1988).Development of a brief coping checklist for use with pediatric populations. *Journal of Pediatric Psychology*, **13**, 555–74.

Spirito, A., Stark, L. J., Williams, C., Stamoulis, D. & Alexon, D. (1988). Coping strategies utilized by referred and non-referred patients and a healthy control group. Poster presented at the Society of Behavioral Medicine Annual Meeting, Boston MA.

Spivack, G. & Shure, M. B. (1982). The cognition of social adjustment: Interpersonal cognitive problem-solving thinking. In B. B. Lahey & A. E. Kazdin (eds.), *Advances in Clinical Child Psychology*, Vol. 5. New York: Plenum Press, pp. 323–72.

(1985). ICPS and beyond: Centripetal and centrifugal forces. *American Journal of Community Psychology*, **13**, 226–43.

Stabler, B. (1988). Pediatric consultation-liaison. In D. K. Routh (ed.), *Handbook of Pediatric Psychology*. New York: Guilford Press, pp. 538–66.

Starfield, B. (1985). The state of research on chronically ill children. In N. Hobbs & J. M. Perrin (eds.), *Issues in the Care of Children with Chronic Illness*. San Francisco: Jossey-Bass, pp. 109–32.

Stehbens, J. A. (1988). Childhood cancer. In D. Routh (ed.), *Handbook of Pediatric Psychology*. New York: Guilford Press, pp. 135–61.

Stehbens, J. A., Kisker, C. T. & Wilson, B. K. (1983). Achievement and intelligence test–retest performance in pediatric cancer patients at diagnosis and one year later. *Journal of Pediatric Psychology*, **8**, 47–56.

Stein, E. K. & Jessop, D. J. (1984). Psychological adjustment among children with chronic conditions. *Pediatrics*, **73**, 169–74.

Steinhausen, H. C. (1976). Hemophilia: A psychological study in chronic disease in juveniles. *Journal of Psychosomatic Research*, **20**, 461–7.

Steinhausen, J. (1982). Locus of control among psychosomatically and chronically ill children and adolescents. *Journal of Abnormal Child Psychology*, **10**, 609–16.

Steward, M. S. & Steward, D. S. (1981). Children's conceptions of medical procedures. In R. Bibace & M. Walsh (eds.), *Children's Conceptions of Health, Illness and Bodily Functions*. San Francisco: Jossey-Bass, pp. 67–84.

Strodtbeck, F. (1951). Husband–wife interaction over revealed differences. *American Sociology Review*, **16**, 468–73.

Swisher, J. D. (1976). Mental Health: The care of preventive health education. *Journal of School Health*, **46**, 386–91.

Tavormina, J. F., Boll, T. J., Dunn, N. J., Luscomb, R. L. & Taylor, J. R. (1981). Psychosocial effects on parents of raising a physically handicapped child. *Journal of Abnormal Child Psychology*, **9**, 121–31.

Taylor, H. G., Albo, V. C., Phebus, C. K., Sachs, B. R. & Bierl, P. G. (1987). Postirradiation treatment outcomes for children with acute lymphocytic leukemia: Clarification of risks. *Journal of Pediatric Psychology*, **12**, 395–412.

Taylor, M. R. H. & O'Connor, P. (1989). Resident parents and shorter hospital stay. *Archives of Disease in Psychology*, **64**, 274–6.

Tesler, M., Ward, J., Savedra, M. Wegner, C. B. & Gibbons, P. (1983). Developing an instrument for eliciting children's descriptions of pain. *Perceptual and Motor Skills*, **56**, 315–21.

Tew, B. & Laurence, K. M. (1973). Mothers, brothers and sisters of patients with spina bifida. *Developmental Medicine and Child Neurology*, **15**, 69–76.

 (1976). The effects of admission to hospital surgery on children with spina bifida. *Developmental Medicine and Child Neurology*, **18** (Suppl. 7), 119–35.

Tew, B. J., Payne, H. & Laurence, K. M. (1974). Must a family with a handicapped child be a handicapped family? *Developmental Medicine and Child Neurology*, **16**, 95–8.

Thornes, R. (1983). Parental access and family facilities in children's wards in England. *British Medical Journal*, **287**, 190–2.

Tin, L. G. & Teasdale, G. R. (1985). An observational study of the social adjustment of spina bifida children in integrated settings. *British Journal of Educational Psychology*, **55**, 81–3.

Turnbull, A. P. & Winton, P. (1983). A comparison of specialized and mainstreamed preschools from the perspectives of parents of handicapped children. *Journal of Pediatric Psychology*, **8**, 57–72.

Ungerer, J., Horgan, B., Chaitow, J. & Champion, G. B. (1988). Psychosocial functioning in children and young adults with juvenile arthritis. *Journal of Pediatrics*, **81**, 195–202.

Varni, J. W. (1983). *Clinical Behavioral Pediatrics: An Interdisciplinary Approach*. New York: Pergamon Press.

Varni, J. W. & Jay, S. M. (1984). Biobehavioural factors in juvenile rheumatoid arthritis: Implications for research and practice. *Clinical Psychology Review*, **4**, 543–50.

Varni, J. W. & Wallander, J. L. (1988). Pediatric chronic disabilities: Hemophilia and spina bifida as examples. In D. Routh (ed.), *Handbook of Pediatric Psychology*. New York: Guilford Press, pp. 190–221.

van der Veer, A. H. (1949). The psychopathology of physical illness and hospital residence. *Quarterly Journal of Child Behavior*, **1**, 55–71.

van Westervelt, D., Brantley, J. & Ware, W. (1983). Changing children's attitudes toward physically handicapped peers: Effects of a film and teacher-led discussion. *Journal of Pediatric Psychology*, **8**, 327–44.

van Westervelt, D. & McKinney, J. D. (1980). Effects of a film on non-handicapped children's attitudes toward handicapped children. *Exceptional Children*, **46**, 294.

Vernon, D. T. A. & Bailey, W. (1974). The use of motion pictures in the psychological preparation of children for induction of anesthesia. *Anesthesiology*, **40**, 68–72.

Vernon, D. T., Foley, J. M., Sipowicz, R. R. & Schulman, J. L. (1965). *The Psychological Responses of Children to Hospitalization and Illness: A Review of the Literature*. Springfield, IL: Thomas.

Visintainer, M. A. & Wolfer, J. A. (1975). Psychological preparation for surgical pediatric patients: The effect on children's and parents' stress responses and adjustment. *Pediatrics*, **56**, 187–202.

Voeltz, L. M. (1982). Effects of structured interactions with severely handicapped peers on children's attitudes. *American Journal of Mental Deficiency*, **86**, 380–90.

Waechter, E. (1971). Children's awareness of fatal illness. *American Journal of Nursing*, **71**, 1168–72.

Waisbren, S. (1980). Parents' reactions to the birth of a developmentally disabled infant. *American Journal of Mental Deficiency*, **84**, 356–61.

Walker, L. S., Ford, M. B. & Donald, W. D. (1986). Stress in families with cystic fibrosis. Paper presented at the annual meeting of the APA, Washington, DC.

Wallander, J. L., Feldman, W. S. & Varni, J. W. (1989). Disease severity and psychosocial adaptation in children with spina bifida. *Journal of Pediatric Psychology*, **14**, 89–102.

Wallander, J. L., Pitt, L. C. & Mellins, C. A. (1990). Risk factors for maladaptation in mothers of physically or sensory handicapped children: Disability status, functional independence, and psychosocial stress. *Journal of Consulting and Clinical Pathology* (in press).

Wallander, J. L. & Varni, J. W. (1986, March). Psychosocial factors, adaptation, and bleeding episodes in hemophilic children. Paper presented at the meeting of the Society of Behavioral Medicine, San Francisco.

Wallander, J. L., Varni, J. W., Babani, L., Banis, H. T., DeHeen, C. B. & Wilcox, K. T. (1989). *Journal of Pediatric Psychology*, **14**, 23–42.

Wallander, J. L., Varni, J. W., Babani, L., Banis, H. T. & Wilcox, K. T. (1988). Children with chronic physical disorders: Maternal reports of their psychological adjustment. *Journal of Pediatric Psychology*, **13**, 197–212.

Wallander, J. L., Varni, J. W., Babani, L., DeHeen, C. B., Wilcox, K. T. & Banis, H. T. (1989). The social environment and the adaptation of mothers of physically handicapped children. *Journal of Pediatric Psychology*, **14**, 371–88.

Walter, C. A. (1986). *The Timing of Motherhood: Is Later Better?* New York: Heath.

Wanschura, T. & Loschenkohl, E. (1979). The child in the hospital: Two models of conditions contributing to reinforcement/inhibition of behavior disorders. *Praxis der Kinderpsychologie und Kinderpsychiatrie*, **28**, 51–5.

Wasserman, A. L., Thompson, E. L. & Wilimas, J. A. (1987). The psychological status of survivors of childhood/adolescent Hodgkin's disease. *Archives of Disease in Childhood*, **141**, 636–31.

Wertlieb, D., Hauser, S. T. & Jacobson, A. (1986). Adaptation to diabetes: Behavior symptoms and family context. *Journal of Pediatric Psychology*, **11**, 463–80.

Wheeler, K., Keiper, A. D., Janoun, L. & Chessells, J. M. (1988). Medical cost of curing childhood acute lymphoblastic leukaemia. *British Medical Journal*, **296**, 162–6.

White, E., Elsom, B. & Prawat, R. (1978). Children's conceptions of death. *Child Development*, **49**, 307–10.

Whiting, B. B. & Edwards, C. P. (1988). *Children of Different Worlds: The Formation of Social Behavior*. Cambridge, MA: Harvard University Press.

Whitt, J. K., Dykstra, W. & Taylor, C. A. (1979). Children's conceptions of illness and cognitive development. *Clinical Pediatrics*, **18**, 327–39.

Wikler, L., Wasow, M. & Hatfield, E. (1981). Chronic sorrow revisited: Parent vs. professional depiction of the adjustment of parents of mentally rearded children. *American Journal of Orthopsychiatry*, **5**, 63–70.

Williams, T., Wetton, N. & Moon, A. (1988). 'Jugs and herrings'. HEC Primary School Project. University of Southampton.

Williamson, P. S. & Williamson, M. L. (1983). Physiologic stress reduction by a local anesthetic during newborn circumcision. *Pediatrics*, **71**, 36–40.

Wills, T. A. (1986). Stress and coping in early adolescence: Relationships to substance use in urban school samples. *Health Psychology*, **5**, 503–29.

Wing, R. R., Lamparski, D. M., Zaslow, S., Betschart, J., Siminerio, L. & Becker, D. (1985). Frequency and accuracy of self-monitoring of blood glucose in children: Relationship to glycemic control. *Diabetes Care*, **8**, 214–18.

Wolfer, J. A. & Visintainer, M. A. (1979). Prehospital psychological preparation for tonsillectomy patients: Effects on children's and parents' adjustment. *Pediatrics*, **64**, 646–55.

Woolf, A., Rappaport, L., Reardon, P., Ciborowski, J., D'Angelo, E. & Bessette, J. (1989). School functioning and disease severity in boys with hemophilia. *Journal of Developmental and Behavioral Pediatrics*, **10**, 81–5.

Worchel, F. F., Nolan, B. F., Willson, V. L., Purcer, J. S., Copeland, D. & Pfefferbaum, B. (1988). Assessment of depression in children with cancer. *Journal of Pediatric Psychology*, **13**, 101–12.

Wortman, C. B. & Silver, R. C. (1987). Coping with irrevocable loss. In G. R. VandenBos & B. K. Bryant (eds.), *Cataclysms, Crises, and Catastrophies: Psychology in Action*. Washington, DC: American Psychological Association, pp. 185–235.

Wright, B. A. (1983). *Physical Disability: A Psychosocial Approach* (2nd edn). New York: Harper & Row.

Zastowny, T. R., Kirschenbaum, D. S. & Meng, A. L. (1986). Coping skills training for children: Effects on distress before, during, and after hospitalization for surgery. *Health Psychology*, **5**, 231–47.

Zeltzer, L. (1980). The adolescent with cancer. In J. Kellerman (ed.), *Psychological Aspects of Childhood Cancer*. Springfield, IL: Thomas.

Zeltzer, L. & LeBaron, S. (1982). Hypnosis and non-hypnotic techniques for reduction of pain and anxiety during painful procedures in children and adolescents with cancer. *Journal of Pediatrics*, **101**, 1032–5.

Author index

Abbott, N. C., 22, 128
Ablin, A., 80, 130
Abu-Saad, H., 31, 128
Achenbach, T., 46, 58, 128
Ack, M., 53, 128
Acosta, P. B., 61, 128
Adler, R., 59, 143
Affleck, G., 97, 128
Agle, D. P., 102, 145
Aisenberg, R. B., 16, 128
Albo, V. C., 51, 155
Alexander, A. B., 97, 128
Alexander, B., 94, 137
Alexon, D., 110, 154
Allen, D. A., 29, 97, 128, 152
Allen, L., 58, 128
Altieri, M. F., 79, 138
Altschuler, A., 21, 128
Anderson, B. J., 53, 128
Anderson, H. R., 49, 58, 67, 128
Anderson, I., 50, 147
Andrasik, F., 30, 129
Anhsjo, S., 53, 129
Anthony, E. J., 137
Appley, M. H., 143
Argyris, C., 98, 129
Armstrong, R. W., 101, 129, 151
Asher, S. R., 123, 149
Atkinson, S., 113, 137
Attanasio, V., 30, 129
Authier, K., 146
Azarnoff, P., 15, 26, 129, 139

Babani, L., 58, 62, 64, 66, 67, 156
Bacon, G., 53, 128
Bailey, P. A., 49, 58, 67, 128

Bailey, W., 23, 155
Baillargeon, R., 89, 118, 137
Baker, B., 34, 37, 131
Baker, L., 75, 147
Bakwin, H., 49, 129
Bakwin, R., 49, 129
Baluk, U., 72, 129
Band, E., 37, 106, 129
Bane, M. J., 77, 129
Banion, J. R., 63, 77, 129
Banis, H. T., 58, 62, 64, 66, 67, 156
Barbarin, O. A., 80, 132
Barbera-Stein, L., 98, 120
Barbour, L., 73, 144
Barclay, C., 53, 128
Barr, R., 35, 129
Barrios, B. A., 23, 33, 129
Bartel, N., 52, 149
Battjes, R., 130, 136
Baum, J. D., 67, 82, 129, 145
Beales, J. G., 84, 129
Beardslee, W., 22, 39, 144
Beck, A. L., 56, 129
Becker, D., 82, 134, 157
Bell, C. S., 130, 136
Bellak, L., 140
Berndt, T. R., 90, 137
Bernstein, A. C., 86, 129
Bessette, J., 54, 157
Betschart, J., 82, 134, 157
Beyer, J. E., 31, 130
Bibace, R., 84, 85, 87, 89, 118, 130, 133,
    142, 146, 154
Bierl, P. G., 51, 155
Billings, A. G., 55, 130
Billings, A. H., 74, 134

Binger, C., 80, 130
Birleson, P., 46, 130
Bloch, S., 67, 145
Blos, P., 93, 130
Blotcky, A. D., 43, 102, 130
Bluebond-Langner, M., 80, 87, 130
Boll, T. J., 61, 66, 75, 130, 154
Bolstad, C. H., 75, 130
Bond, L. A., 87, 151
Boone, R. R., 20, 151
Borner, A., 62, 130
Botvin, G. J., 98, 99, 130
Bowlby, J., 14, 72, 131
Boyle, M., 42, 48, 120, 132
Bradbury, J. A., 101, 131
Brantley, J., 101, 156
Breslau, N., 47, 57, 61, 62, 73, 131
Brett, A., 18, 131
Brewer, E., 54, 141
Brewster, A. B., 13, 87, 131
Brink, S., 43, 75, 102, 139
Britton, J. R., 101, 140
Brody, G. H., 73, 131
Brookhauser, T., 146
Brown, A. L., 89, 131
Brown, J. M., 34, 37, 131
Brown, R., 53, 136
Brownlee-Duffeck, M., 18, 23, 149
Bruhn, J. G., 54, 131
Bryant, B. K., 157
Buchanan, D. G., 46, 130
Burbach, D. J., 35, 131
Burgert, E. O., 71, 148
Burgmeier, R., 27, 152
Burke, E. J., 30, 129
Burns, W. J., 21, 143
Burr, C. K., 43, 102, 132
Bush, J. P., 25, 132
Butler, E., 68, 145

Cadman, D., 42, 48, 120, 132
Cairns, N., 69, 100, 143
Caldwell, H. S., 103, 132
Califano, J. A. Jr, 117, 132
Camitta, B. M., 63, 83, 147
Campbell, M. M., 57, 139
Candee, D., 75, 133
Carey, S., 89, 118, 132
Carey, W. B., 129
Carpenter, P. J., 70, 71, 147

Carr, A., 137
Carson, K. L., 79, 145
Carter, A., 68, 142
Carter, M. C., 63, 77, 129
Carver, C. S., 106, 108, 110, 115, 132
Cassell, S., 22, 38, 132
Cederblad, M., 75, 139
Cervero, F., 147
Chadwick, M. W., 99, 141
Chaitow, J., 55, 58, 59, 155
Champion, G. B., 55, 58, 59, 155
Champion, L. A. A., 79, 138
Chan, J. M., 22, 132
Chandler, B. C., 54, 131
Chapman, J., 31, 33, 146
Chesler, M. A., 80, 103, 132
Chess, S., 132
Chessells, J. M., 51, 157
Chi, M. T. H., 90, 132
Chodoff, P., 71, 132
Christensen, N., 81, 145
Christopherson, E. R., 93, 150
Ciborowski, J., 54, 157
Citrin, W. B., 99, 100, 136
Claerhout, S., 117, 132
Clark, M. W., 57, 142
Clarke, D. W., 82, 153
Clarke, M. S., 144
Clarson, C., 82, 132
Clemente, I., 94, 151
Close, H., 53, 133
Clunies-Ross, C., 88, 133
Cohen, L. H., 110, 138
Colby, A., 75, 133
Collier, G., 81, 133
Collins, W. A., 125, 133, 145
Compas, B. E., 44, 110, 133
Contento, I. R., 84, 147
Connell, D. B., 100, 133
Consumers Association, 16, 133
Cooper, J. A., 49, 58, 67, 128
Copeland, D. R., 51, 63, 83, 144, 157
Costa, P. T. Jr, 86, 108, 142, 145
Cousens, P., 51, 133
Cowan, P. A., 86, 129
Cos, D. J., 94, 149
Craig, K. D., 31, 133, 138
Crain, A., 69, 133
Crawford, P., 73, 104, 134
Creet, T. L., 49, 50, 94, 133, 151

Crider, C., 85, 133
Crisco, J. J., 63, 83, 147
Crittenden, M., 101, 133
Crittenden, M. R., 56, 129
Crocker, A. C., 73, 129, 134
Crocker, E., 21, 134
Crouse-Novak, M., 70, 143
Crowl, M., 22, 134
Culling, J., 88, 142
Cunningham, S. J., 30, 131
Cuskey, W., 54, 144

Dahl, R., 12, 134
Daneman, D., 82, 132, 134
D'Angelo, E., 54, 157
Daniels, D., 74, 134
Danowski, T. S., 53, 143
Dash, J., 39, 136
Davenport, S. L. H., 57, 139
Davies, A. G., 53, 133
Debuskey, M., 88, 134
De Heen, C. B., 62, 64, 66, 156
de la Suta, A., 95, 144
De Loache, J. S., 89, 131
De Longis, A., 106, 136
Dennis, B., 134
Desmond, K., 62, 83, 95, 148
Dias, J. K., 79, 148
Dimond, M. E., 16, 152
Domino, E., 75, 130
Donald, W. D., 66, 156
Dorner, S., 57, 134
Douglas, J., 14, 134
Drash, A., 53, 58, 82, 134, 152
Drotar, D., 73, 104, 127, 134
Dubner, R., 146
Duffy, E., 33, 134
Dunbar, J., 93, 134
Dunkel-Schetter, C., 106, 136
Dunn, E. G., 34, 35, 137
Dunn, J., 5, 31, 33, 74, 134, 146
Dunn, N. J., 61, 66, 75, 154
Dweck, C. S., 113, 114, 134, 135
Dykstra, W., 84, 87, 157

Easson, W., 135
Edelbrook, C., 46, 58, 128
Edwards, C. P., 124, 157
Ehrlich, R. M., 53, 58, 82, 132, 151

Eiser, C., 12, 19, 21, 35, 43, 51, 61, 82,
    84, 87, 91, 95, 97, 98, 100, 101, 113,
    135
Eiser, J. R., ix, 87, 91, 98, 100, 135, 144
Eisler, R. M., 152
Elkins, P. D., 18, 20, 21, 135, 136, 151
Ellenberg, L., 39, 136
Elliott, C. H., 31, 32, 33, 40, 41, 136, 141
Ellis, E. F., 153
Elsom, B., 86, 157
Erhlich, R. M., 132
Erikson, E., 59, 136
Ernst, N., 134
Etzwiler, D. D., 81, 94, 133, 136
Evans, A., 80 136
Evans, W. S., 94, 149

Fairclough, D., 51, 52, 124, 147
Faust, D., 73, 74, 145
Feinberg, T. L., 70, 142
Feldman, W. S., 57, 156
Ferguson, B. F., 136
Ferguson, D. M., 16, 23, 152
Ferrari, M., 73, 136
Feuerstein, R., 80, 130
Fiedler, J. L., 61, 128
Field, T., 33, 136
Fields, H. L., 146
Fine, R., 98, 142
Finkelstein, R., 70, 142
Firestone, P., 128
Fischman, S. E., 70, 141
Fiske, S. T., 144
Flanagan, J., 96, 136
Flavell, J. H., 138, 145
Flay, B. R., 98, 136
Fochtman, D., 71, 143
Foley, J. M., 17, 155
Folkins, C. H., 87, 148
Folkman, S., 105, 106, 136, 144
Follansbee, D. J., 75, 76, 99, 100, 136,
    139
Fonagny, P., 53, 136
Fondacaro, K. M., 110, 133
Forbes, C., 53, 54, 145
Ford, M. B., 66, 156
Foster, D. J., 80, 153
Fowler, M., 113, 137
Frank, M., 82, 132
Franks, C. M., 146

Freund, A., 94, 137
Friedman, A. G., 52, 124, 147
Friedman, S. B., 54, 62, 71, 98, 132, 137, 139, 145
Fritz, G. K., 124, 137
Furman, A. E., 87, 137
Futterman, E., 70, 137

Gaffney, A., 34, 35, 137
Gagnon-Lefebvre, B., 26, 151
Gamble, W., 73, 146
Ganofsky, M. A., 104, 134
Garbarino, J., 146
Garber, J., 135, 153
Garmezy, N., 75, 137, 141, 144
Garner, A. M., 81, 137
Garralda, M. E., 56, 137
Garvey, C., 90, 137
Gath, A., 69, 137
Gayton, W. F., 62, 137
Gellert, E., 85, 86, 130, 137
Gelman, R., 89, 118, 137
Gerrity, P. S., 59, 80, 84, 118, 149
Gershaw, N. J., 98, 138
Giannini, E., 54, 141
Gibbons, P., 33, 152, 155
Gibbs, J., 75, 133
Gilbert, B., 95, 138
Gilchrist, G. S., 71, 148
Ginther, L. J., 20, 151
Glaser, R., 90, 132
Glick, B., 98, 138
Gluck, R. S., 79, 138
Glynn, T., 130
Glyshaw, K., 110, 138
Gochman, D., 36, 138
Godfrey, S., 50, 148
Gofman, H., 101, 133
Golden, M. P., 53, 138
Goldstein, A. P., 98, 138, 146
Goldstein, G., 53, 128
Goldson, E., 33, 136
Gonder-Frederick, L., 94, 149
Goodman, J. R., 31, 33, 146
Goodyer, I. M., 53, 133
Gortmaker, S. L., 138
Goslin, E. R., 21, 27, 138
Gottlieb, J. E., 55, 130
Graham, P. J., 48, 49, 66, 120, 138, 151
Grant Foundation, William T., 149

Gray, D. L., 53, 138
Greene, P., 101, 138
Greenbaum, P. E., 25, 132
Greenberg, H. S., 52, 138
Greenberg, L. W., 79, 138
Gresham, F. M., 46, 56, 144
Greundel, J., 90, 148
Greydanus, D. E., 98, 138
Grgic, M. D., 82, 145
Grobstein, R., 70, 141
Gross, A. M., 99, 112, 138
Gross, R. T., 129
Grossman, F. K., 73, 138
Gruen, R., 106, 136
Grunau, R. V. E., 31, 138
Gualtieri, T., 124, 139
Guetz, T. E., 114, 134
Gurwich, R., 42, 102, 130
Gustafson, P. A., 75, 139
Guylay, J.-E., 100, 143

Hagen, J., 53, 128
Hall, L. J., 73, 144
Hamburg, D. A., 71, 132
Hampton, J. W., 54, 131
Haney, J. I., 117, 141
Hansell, S., 36, 146
Hansen, C. A., 94, 137
Hansen, P., 22, 128
Hanson, K., 29, 152
Hanson, L., 19, 135
Hardy, S., 62, 83, 95, 148
Harkavy, J., 62, 82, 83, 92, 93, 95, 117, 139, 141
Harm, D. L., 50, 133
Harpin, V. A., 33, 139
Harrison, C. W., 49, 150
Harter, S., 46, 139
Hartman, D., 33, 129
Hartup, W. W., 74, 109, 133, 139
Hasazi, J. E., 87, 151
Hassanein, R., 69, 143
Hatfield, E., 72, 157
Hauser, S., 43, 75, 76, 102, 139, 156
Hayden, P. W., 57, 139
Heckhausen, J., 125, 139
Heffernan, M., 26, 139
Heiligstein, E., 123, 139
Heisler, A. B., 98, 139
Heller, A., 51, 140

Hellrung, I., 82, 145
Herlich, R., 62, 83, 95, 148
Hersen, M., 152
Herskowitz, R. D., 75, 76, 139
Herz, E. J., 98, 140
Hester, N. K., 30, 140
Heston, J. V., 94, 140
Hetherington, E. M., 139
Hewer, A., 75, 133
Hewins, J., 56, 129
Hicks, R. E., 124, 139
Higgins, G., 39, 136
Hilgard, J. K., 39, 140, 144
Hilgard, J. R., 39, 140
Hill, R. A., 49, 101, 140
Hirsch, B., 68, 140
Hoagland, A. C., 70, 71, 147
Hoare, P., 62, 140
Hobbs, N., 42, 49, 132, 138, 140, 146, 154
Hoffman, I., 70, 98, 137, 138
Hollandsworth, J. G. Jr, 26, 150
Holmes, F. F., 124, 140
Holmes, H. A., 124, 140
Holt, P. J. L., 84, 129
Honig, G., 71, 143
Hoppe, M., 53, 58, 151
Hops, H., 45, 140
Horgan, B., 55, 58, 59, 155
Horowitz, M. J., 72, 140
Houlihan, J., 75, 76, 139
Hudson, I., 46, 130
Humble, Y., 53, 129
Humner, K. M., 53, 138
Humphreys, P., 30, 151
Hunt, J., 87, 135
Hurtig, A. L., 56, 58, 124, 140
Hynes, P., 87, 148

Ingalls, A., 88, 140
Ingersoll, G. M., 53, 138
Inhelder, B., 59, 150
Ivey, J., 54, 141

Jackson, J., 147
Jacobs, A. M., 94, 96, 109, 146
Jacobson, A., 43, 75, 76, 102, 139, 156
Jacobson, P. B., 123, 139
Jameson, R. A., 56, 137
Janoun, L., 51, 157

Jay, S. M., 31–3, 40, 41, 117, 136, 141, 155
Jessop, D. J., 58, 154
Jewett, L. S., 79, 138
Johnson, G., 31, 33, 146
Johnson, M., 113, 137
Johnson, S. B., 53, 62, 82, 83, 92–5, 117, 137–9, 141
Johnson, W. G., 99, 112, 138
Johnston, C. C., 33, 141
Jones, R. T., 117, 141

Kagan, J., 109, 141
Kagen, L. B., 98, 141
Kandt, R., 53, 128
Kaltreider, N. B., 72, 140
Kaplan, D. M., 70, 141
Kaplan, M., 95, 144
Kaplan, R. M., 99, 141
Karasu, T., 140
Karoly, P., 118, 141
Karon, M., 80, 88, 153
Kashani, J. H., 50, 59, 141
Kastenbaum, R., 86, 142
Katz, E. R., 31, 33, 41, 101, 141, 142
Katz, R. M., 50, 153
Kaufer, F. H., 146
Kauffmann, K., 75, 133
Kazak, A. E., 52, 57, 68, 138, 142
Kazdin, A. E., 117, 131, 141, 142, 154
Keen, J. H., 84, 129
Keiper, A. D., 51, 157
Kellerman, J., 31, 39, 101, 136, 142, 153, 158
Kelley, M. L., 46, 56, 144
Kendrick, C., 88, 142
Keneally, T., 12, 142
King, E. H., 61, 142
King, S. M., 101, 129, 151
Kirschenbaum, D. S., 24, 26, 157
Kisker, C. T., 100, 154
Kjellman, N. I. M., 75, 139
Klein, R. H., 103, 148
Klinzing, D. G., 20, 142
Klinzing, D. R., 20, 142
Koch, P., 109, 153
Koch, R., 61, 128
Koenig, P., 50, 59, 141
Koepke, D., 56, 140
Kohlberg, L., 75, 133

Koocher, G. P., 70, 71, 79, 80, 86, 142, 153
Korsch, B. M., 98, 142
Koupernick, C., 137
Kovacs, M., 46, 70, 142
Krohne, H. W., 135
Kubany, A. J., 53, 143
Kubler-Ross, E., 72, 143
Kupst, M. J., 70, 71, 143, 148
Kurtz, A. B., 53, 135
Kushner, J., 80, 130
Kutscher, A., 137
Kuttner, L., 39, 40, 143

Lacey, J. I., 33, 143
La Greca, A. M., 93, 97, 99, 100, 136, 143
Lahey, B. B., 131, 154
Lamb, M. E., 74, 143
Lamb, W., 103, 152
Lamparski, D. M., 82, 157
Lancaster, S., 59, 143
Landau, L. I., 82, 95, 145
Lane, D. M., 103, 132
Lang, J., 91, 135
Lansdown, R., 88, 133
Lansky, S., 69, 100, 143
Larsson, G., 53, 129
Laurence, K. M., 57, 62, 69, 73, 143, 155
Laux, L., 135
Lavigne, J. V., 21, 143
Lazar, S. J., 94, 140
Lazarus, R. S., 105, 106, 136, 143, 144
Le Baron, S., 39, 40, 140, 144, 158
Lei, T., 68, 145
Leibman, R., 75, 147
Leiderman, P. H., 109, 144
Leikin, S. L., 79, 138
Lemanek, K. L., 46, 56, 144
Leonard, R. L., 24, 26, 153
Letovsky, E., 94, 151
Leukeveld, C., 130
Leung, P., 94, 133
Levenson, P. M., 63, 83, 144
Leventhal, H., 24, 25, 144
Leventhal, J. M., 69, 70, 94, 151, 152
Leveque, K. L., 103, 132
Levin, I., 89, 118, 144
Levine, M. D., 129
Levy, R., 134
Lewis, K., 22, 128

Lewis, C., 34, 36, 95, 117, 144
Lewis, M., 34, 36, 95, 117, 144
Ley, P., 95, 144
Licht, B. G., 113, 135
Lindsay, M. K. M., 53, 136
Lindemann, J. E., 80, 144
Lineberger, H. O., 144
Link, J., 82, 132
Linn, S., 22, 38, 39, 144
Lipnick, R. N., 79, 138
Lipowski, Z. J., 46, 120, 144
Lipsitt, L. P., 46, 144
Litt, I., 54, 144
Lloyd, B. B., 151
Lobato, D., 73, 74, 144, 145
Lorenz, R., 81, 145
Loschenkohl, E., 16, 156
Lowman, J. T., 69, 100, 143
Ludvigsson, J., 75, 139
Luscomb, R. L., 61, 66, 75, 154
Lutzker, J. R., 117, 132

Maccoby, E. E., 125, 145
MacDonald, K., 53, 54, 145
MacLean, E. W., 99, 149
MacLean, W. E., 50, 66, 149
MacLean, W. E., Jr, 48, 149
Madden, N. A., 54, 145
Maddux, J. E., 117, 145
Malcarne, V. L., 110, 133
Malone, J., 82, 145
Malpas, J. S., 51, 145
Malphus, E., 82, 145
Mandler, J., 89, 118, 145
Marion, R. J., 50, 133
Markman, E. M., 138, 145
Markova, I., 53, 54, 145
Marrero, O., 52, 149
Marsh, E. J., 129
Marshall, I. A., 57, 131
Marteau, T. M., 67, 145
Martin, A. J., 82, 95, 145
Mason, E. F., 100, 133
Mattson, A. E., 75, 102, 130, 145
Maurer, H., 71, 143
McAlister, R., 68, 145
McAnarney, E. R., 54, 145
McAndrew, I., 57, 145
McCallum, M., 62, 82, 83, 92, 93, 95, 117, 138, 139, 141
McCarthy, C. A., 71, 148

McCarthy, P., 94, 151
McCrae, R. R., 108, 145
McDonald, A. C., 79, 145
McFadden, E. R., Jr, 60, 146
McGarvey, M. E., 18, 146
McGrade, B. K., 97, 128
McGrath, P. J., 29–31, 33, 34, 117, 128, 146, 151
McHale, S., 73, 101, 146
McKinney, J. D., 101, 157
McMahon, R. J., 31, 133
McNabb, W. L., 94, 96, 109, 146
Meadows, A. T., 52, 138, 149
Mearig, J. S., 43, 113, 146
Mechanic, D., 34, 36, 146
Meichenbaum, D., 23, 24, 146
Meijer, A., 62, 146
Melamed, B. G., 23, 25, 132, 146
Mellins, C. A., 63, 65, 156
Mellor, V. P., 84, 129
Meltzer, J., 87, 146
Melzack, R., 30, 33, 147
Meng, A. L., 24, 26, 157
Merskey, H., 29, 147
Messenger, K., 73, 131
Michela, J. L., 84, 147
Middleton, E., Jr, 153
Mikkelsen, C., 80, 130
Miles, M. S., 63, 77, 129
Miller, C. T., 73, 144
Miller, D. J., 27, 149
Miller, I., 53, 128
Miller, J., 54, 147
Miller, J. J. III, 55, 74, 130, 134
Miller, P. M., 152
Miller, S., 36, 108, 147
Milman, L., 75, 147
Milunsky, A., 134
Minuchin, S., 75, 147
Mitchell, R., 68, 147
Mongeon, M., 26, 151
Montagner, H., 109, 153
Moon, A., 100, 157
Moore, S. L., 46, 56, 144
Moos, B. S., 67, 147
Moos, R. G., 67, 147
Moos, R. H., 55, 74, 130, 134
Moran, G. S., 53, 136
Morgan, A. H., 39, 140
Morgan, E., 71, 143
Morgan, S. A., 147

Morgan, S. B., 75, 153
Mori, L., 21, 27, 149
Morison, J. D., 31, 133
Morris, D. A., 50, 59, 141
Morrow, G. R., 70, 71, 147
Morrow, J. R., 63, 83, 144
Mortimer, E. A., 47, 131
Moses, C., 53, 143
Mott, M., 88, 142
Mrazek, D. A., 50, 147
Mulhern, R. K., 51, 52, 63, 83, 124, 147
Mullett, M., 99, 112, 138
Mussen, P. H., 139
Myers, B. A., 79, 148
Myers-Vando, R., 87, 148

Nadas, A. S., 16, 128
Nader, P. R., 94, 148
Natapoff, J., 84, 87, 148
Negrette, V. G., 98, 142
Nelson, K., 89, 90, 91, 118, 148
Nethercut, G. E., 56, 129
Nimorwicz, P., 103, 148
Noam, G., 76, 139
Nolan, B. F., 51, 157
Nolan, T., 62, 83, 95, 148
Norrish, M., 50, 148
Novak, D., 80, 148
Nowicki, S., 46, 148

Oakhill, T., 88, 142
Obetz, S. W., 71, 148
Ochs, J., 51, 147
O'Connor, P., 16, 155
Offord, D. R., 42, 48, 120, 122
Ogle, P. A., 73, 150
O'Grady, D. J., 141
O'Keeffe, J., 34, 37, 131
Olch, D., 54, 148
Olness, K., 39, 148
Olson, R., 40, 141
O'Malley, J. E., 70, 71, 80, 142, 153
O'Neill, P., 72, 129
Orford, J., 135
Orr, D. P., 57, 148
Ozolins, M., 40, 141

Palmer, D. J., 79, 145
Palmer, J. S., 49, 58, 67, 128
Pantell, R. H., 79, 148
Parcel, G. S., 94, 148

Paris, J., 80, 132
Park, K. B., 56, 140
Parker, J. G., 123, 149
Partridge, J. W., 81, 137
Patenaude, A. F., 22, 39, 144
Patterson, D., 12, 61, 97, 135
Paul, M., 22, 132
Paulauskas, S., 70, 142
Payne, H., 69, 155
Peckham, V. C., 52, 149
Pendergast, J. F., 82, 153
Pentz, M. A., 98, 149
Pennebaker, J. W., 94, 149
Peretz, D., 137
Perlman, K., 82, 132
Perrin, E. C., 44, 50, 59, 66, 80, 84, 118, 149
Perrin, J. M., 42, 48–50, 66, 99, 132, 138, 140, 146, 149, 154
Peshkin, M. M., 50, 149
Peterson, C., 18, 23, 149
Peterson, L., 15, 16, 20, 21, 24–7, 35, 104, 131, 134, 149–51
Pfefferbaum, B., 51, 63, 83, 144, 157
Phebus, C. K., 51, 155
Phelan, P. D., 82, 985, 145
Phillips, C., 14, 150
Piaget, J., 34, 35, 59, 84, 90, 118, 150
Pichert, J., 81, 145
Piers, E. Y., 46, 150
Pinkerton, P., 44–7, 150
Pinto, R. P., 26, 150
Pitt, L. C., 63, 65, 156
Plank, E., 80, 150
Platt Committee, Great Britain, 8, 15, 150
Pless, I. B., 44–9, 51, 54, 57, 120, 138, 140, 145, 148, 150
Plummer, R., 80, 148
Pohl, S., 94, 149
Pollak, T., 62, 82, 83, 95, 141
Pollock, M., 70, 142
Porter, C., 86, 150
Postlethwaite, J. R., 56, 137
Potter, P. C., 87, 150
Powell, T. H., 73, 150
Power, C., 75, 133
Powers, S., 76, 139
Prawat, R., 86, 157
Price, D. A., 53, 133

Prior, M., 59, 143
Pruitt, S. D., 40, 141
Purcer, J. S., 51, 157

Quinton, D., 14, 27, 150

Rachelsefsky, G., 50, 95, 144, 153
Rachman, S., 14, 150
Raczynski, J. M., 43, 102, 130
Rafman, S., 51, 140
Rajapark, D. C., 75, 76, 139
Ramsey, B. K., 44, 149
Rando, R. A., 71, 150
Rapoff, M. A., 93, 150
Rappaport, L., 54, 157
Ratzan, S., 97, 128
Rawls, D. J., 49, 150
Rawls, J. R., 49, 150
Reardon, P., 54, 157
Reber, M., 68, 142
Redpath, C. C., 12, 150
Reed, C. E., 153
Rees, E., 90, 132
Reilly, T. P., 87, 151
Reis, J. S., 98, 140
Reiss, D., 75, 151
Renne, C. M., 49, 151
Repucci, N. D., 114, 135
Reynolds, J. M., 56, 137
Rhymes, J., 24, 26, 153
Richardson, G. M., 30, 151
Ridley-Johnson, R., 15, 20, 21, 27, 149
Rifkind, R., 134
Rigler, D., 80, 88, 101, 142, 153
Robb, J. R., 94, 136
Roberts, M. C., 18, 20, 21, 87, 104, 117, 134–6, 145, 149–51
Robertson, J., 14, 26, 151
Rodabaugh, B., 94, 152
Rodin, J., 21, 151
Rogers, C. S., 12, 150
Roghmann, K. J., 48, 120, 150
Rosch, E., 89, 151
Rosenbaum, M., 146
Rosenbaum, P. L., 101, 129, 151
Rosenberg, A., 54, 144
Rosenbloom, A., 62, 82, 83, 92–5, 117, 138, 139, 141, 145, 153
Rosenblum, E. L., 30, 129
Rosenthal, A., 16, 128

Roskies, E., 26, 151
Rosman, B., 75, 147
Ross, A. W., 79, 148
Ross, D. M., 30, 31, 34, 35, 37, 112, 151
Ross, S. A., 30, 31, 34, 35, 37, 112, 151
Routh, D., 133, 143, 149, 153–5
Rovet, J. F., 53, 58, 151
Rubin, D. H., 94, 151
Russell, B. P., 53, 138
Russell, G., 125, 133
Rutter, M. L., 14, 27, 44, 48, 49, 66, 120,
   137, 138, 141, 144, 150–2
Rutter, N., 33, 139
Ryan, C., 53, 58, 152

Sabbeth, B. F., 69, 70, 152
Sachs, B. R., 51, 155
Sadock, R. T., 94, 151
Said, J., 51, 133
Saille, H., 27, 152
Salerno, M., 88, 140
Salkever, D., 62, 131
Sanders, S. H., 34, 37, 131
Sandler, H. M., 44, 149
Satterwhite B., 54, 57, 145, 148
Saunders, A. M., 103, 152
Savedra, M., 33, 152, 155
Scamagas, P., 94, 152
Schachter, F. F., 134
Schechter, N. L., 29, 152
Scheier, M. F., 106, 108, 110, 115, 132
Schilder, P., 86, 152
Schillinger, J., 31, 33, 146
Schimmel, L. E., 99, 141
Schinke, S. P., 98, 152
Schmidt, L. R., 27, 152
Schoenberg, B., 137
Schottland, P., 94, 151
Schulman, J. L., 17, 70, 71, 143, 148, 155
Schultheis, K., 27, 149
Schwirian, P. M., 73, 152
Sehgman, M. E. P., 135
Seligman, M. E. P., 153
Selman, R. L., 123, 152
Sergis-Deavenport, E., 97, 152
Settergren-Carlsson, G., 53, 129
Shannon, F. T., 16, 152
Shapiro, E. K., 77, 152
Share, L., 79, 80, 152
Sheposh, J. P., 71, 153

Shepperd, J. A., 50, 59, 141
Sheras, P. J., 25, 132
Sherman, M., 98, 138
Shigetomi, C. C., 16, 23–6, 33, 129, 150
Shipp, J. C., 93, 152
Shope, J. T., 97, 153
Shure, M. B., 112, 113, 115, 154
Siegel, S. C., 33, 41, 50, 141, 153
Siegel, S. E., 31, 101, 142
Siegler, R., 131
Silberberg, Y., 63, 83, 144
Silver, R. C., 72, 106, 153, 157
Silverstein, J., 62, 82, 83, 92, 93, 95, 117,
   138, 139, 141, 153
Simeonsson, R. J., 101, 146
Siminerio, L., 82, 134, 157
Simonds, J. F., 98, 153
Simpson, U., 54, 147
Sines, L. K., 81, 136
Sipowicz, R. R., 17, 155
Skipper, J. K., Jr, 24, 26, 153
Slavin, L. A., 80, 153
Slay, T., 79, 145
Sleddon, E. A., 117, 145
Smith, A., 70, 141
Smith, C. W., 101, 131
Smith, K., 43, 102, 130
Smith, R., 80, 148
Soissignan, R., 109, 153
Sourkes, B., 70, 153
Spaulding, B. R., 75, 153
Speicher-Dubin, B., 75, 133
Spencer, R. F., 54, 153
Spillar, R., 62, 82, 83, 92, 93, 95, 117,
   138, 139, 141, 153
Spinetta, J. J., 51, 70, 71, 79, 80, 87, 88,
   103, 134, 153
Spinetta, P., 51, 70, 87, 153
Spirito, A., 73, 74, 110, 111, 115, 145,
   154
Spitz, P., 54, 147
Spivack, G., 112, 113, 115, 154
Sprafkin, R. P., 98, 138
Stabler, B., 127, 154
Stamoulis, D., 110, 154
Standen, P. J., 49, 140
Starfield, B., 45, 154
Stark, L. J., 110, 115, 154
Staruch, K. S., 47, 62, 131
Steffen, J. J., 141

Stehbens, J. A., 51, 100, 154
Stein, E. K., 58, 154
Steinhausen, H. C., 54, 62, 130, 154
Steinhausen, J., 50, 154
Sterky, G., 53, 129
Sternberg, R., 132
Stevens, M., 51, 133
Stevenson, J. E., 147
Steward, D. S., 12, 86, 154
Steward, M. S., 12, 86, 87, 148, 154
Stewart, T. J., 79, 148
Stone, R. K., 134
Stoneman, Z., 73, 131
Strada, M. E., 33, 141
Strauss, N. L., 114, 134
Strickland, B. R., 46, 148
Strodtbeck, F., 75, 154
Strunk, R., 50, 147
Stunkard, A. J., 93, 134
Sugerman, S., 139
Sussman, M., 69, 133
Sutton-Smith, D., 74, 143
Swarner, J. A., 71, 153
Swenson, W. M., 71, 148
Swisher, J. D., 98, 154
Szatmari, P., 42, 48, 120, 122

Tattersfield, A. E., 49, 101, 140
Tavormina, J. B., 61, 66, 75, 154
Tavormina, J. F., 62, 137
Taylor, C. A., 84, 87, 157
Taylor, H. G., 51, 155
Taylor, J. R., 61, 66, 75, 154
Taylor, M. R. H., 16, 155
Teasdale, G. R., 122, 155
Tennen, H., 97, 128
Terdal, L. G., 129
Terrizzi, J., 54, 145
Tesler, M., 33, 152, 155
Tew, B., 57, 62, 69, 73, 143, 155
Thomas, A., 132
Thompson, C. W., 81, 137
Thompson, E. L., 51, 156
Thornes, R., 15, 155
Tiernan, D., 94, 148
Tin, L. G., 122, 155
Tizard, J., 48, 152
Todd, T., 75, 147
Tooley, M., 50, 148
Towbes, L. C., 110, 138

Town, C., 82, 95, 101, 135
Town, R., 61, 97, 135
Tracy, K., 27, 149
Transne, D., 82, 134
Trickett, E., 68, 147
Tripp, J. H., ix, 82, 95, 135
Trumball, R., 143
Tucker, F., 62, 137
Turnbull, A. P., 100, 155
Turner, R. R., 100, 133
Tye, V., 110, 154

Ungerer, J., 55, 58, 59, 155
Unruh, A. M., 29, 30, 34, 117, 146

VandenBos, G. R., 157
van der Veer, A. H., 25, 155
Varni, J. W., 47, 48, 54, 57, 58, 62, 64, 66, 67, 94, 97, 117, 125, 152, 155, 156
Vats, T., 100, 143
Vega, A., 53, 58, 152
Vernon, D. T. A., 17, 23, 155
Visintainer, M. A., 26, 156, 157
Voeltz, L. M., 101, 156

Waechter, E., 88, 156
Waisbren, S., 68, 156
Walker, C. E., 149
Walker, L. S., 66, 156
Wallace, D. B., 77, 152
Wallander, J. L., 47, 48, 54, 57, 58, 62–7, 125, 155, 156
Walsh, M., 84, 85, 87, 89, 118, 130, 133, 142, 146, 154
Walter, C. A., 126, 156
Wanschura, T., 16, 156
Ward, J., 33, 152, 155
Ware, W., 101, 156
Wasow, M., 72, 157
Wasserman, A. L., 51, 52, 124, 147, 156
Waters, B., 51, 133
Weber, F. T., 82, 145
Wechsler, D., 86, 152
Wegner, C., 33, 152, 155
Wehr, J., 69, 143
Weil, W. B., 53, 69, 128
Weill, W., Jr, 133
Weintraub, J. M., 106, 108, 110, 115, 132
Weiss, B., 76, 139
Weiss-Perry, B., 75, 76, 139

Weisz, J. R., 37, 38, 106, 129
Weitzman, M., 73, 131
Weller, S. C., 57, 148
Wells, P., 79, 148
Wentworth, D., 43, 76, 102, 133
Wertlieb, D., 43, 75, 76, 102, 139, 156
van Westervelt, D., 101, 156, 157
West, S., 49, 58, 67, 128
Wetton, N., 100, 157
Wheeler, K., 51, 157
White, E., 86, 157
White, L. S., 56, 58, 124, 140
Whiting, B. B., 124, 157
Whitmore, K., 48, 152
Whitt, J. K., 84, 87, 157
Wikler, L., 72, 157
Wilcox, B., 68, 142
Wilcox, K. T., 58, 62, 64, 66, 67, 156
Wildman, H. E., 99, 112, 138
Wilfley, D., 50, 59, 141
Wilimas, J. A., 51, 156
Williams, C., 110, 115, 154
Williams, G., 54, 147
Williams, J. R., 124, 137
Williams, K. O., 101, 142
Williams, T., 100, 157
Williamson, D. A., 46, 56, 144
Williamson, M. L., 31, 33, 157
Williamson, P. S., 31, 33, 157
Wills, T. A., 98, 110, 130, 157

Willson, V. L., 51, 157
Wilson, B. K., 100, 154
Wilson-Pessano, S. R., 94, 96, 109, 146
Wing, R. R., 82, 157
Winton, P., 100, 155
Wolfer, J. A., 26, 155, 157
Wolfsdorf, J. I., 75, 76, 139
Wolff, P. H., 16, 128
Wolff, S., 46, 130
Wolraich, M., 153
Woody, P., 15, 31, 32, 129, 136
Woolf, A., 54, 157
Worchel, F. F., 51, 157
Wortele, S. K., 20, 151
Wortman, C. B., 72, 106, 113, 135, 153, 157
Wright, B. A., 72, 157
Wright, L., 117, 145
Wunsch, M. G., 94, 149

Yule, W., 48, 49, 66, 120, 1ı38, 151

Zaskow, C., 31, 133
Zaslow, S., 82, 157
Zastowny, T. R., 24, 26, 157
Zeltzer, L., 39, 40, 136, 158
Zigler, E., 58, 128
Zoger, S., 80, 130
Zvagulis, I., 51, 140
Zwartjes, W., 100, 143

Subject index

absence from school, 44, 49, 53, 113
adjustment
  and age, 58, 59
  asthma, 49–51
  birth defects, 51
  cancer, 51–2
  communication and, 80
  coping strategies, *see* coping strategies
  definition, 44–5
  diabetes, 53, 58
  different diseases compared, 57–8
  family, 4, 9, 61–77, 125–6; marital
    relationship, 69–70; resistance
    factors, 67–74; resources, 67–8;
    social support networks, 68–9
  gender, 124
  haemophilia, 53–4, 58
  and informant, 59
  intervention programmes and, 93, 95
  long-term, 124
  marital, 69–70
  maternal, *see* mother
  methodology, 45–6
  outcome measures, 121–3; intelli-
    gence, 121–2; personality, 123;
    social, 122–3
  population-based research, 48–9
  renal disease, 55
  rheumatoid arthritis, 54–5
  risk factors, 64–6
  siblings, 72–4
  sickle-cell anaemia, 56–7
  social support and, 68–9
  spina bifida, 57, 58
  theoretical approaches, 46–8

  and time since diagnosis, 123–4
  types of coping strategy, 110
  see also psychological effects
admission to hospital, 4, 8, 11–27
adolescents, 5–6, 55–7, 76, 97, 124
  self-assessment of health, 36
  social skill teaching, 98–100
  understanding of chronic disease,
    81–3 *passim*
analgesics, 29
anticipatory nausea, 41
anxiety, 17, 21, 26, 33, 53, 62, 80
appraisal, 106
asthma
  adjustment, 49–51
  child's understanding of, 82–3
  family: interactions, 75; resources, 67
  incidence and survival, 2
  intervention programmes, 94, 95–6,
    99–100
  severity, 2–3

birth defects, 51
body, concepts of, 85–6
bone-marrow aspiration, 14, 22, 39, 41
bone-marrow transplants, 22
books, on hospital and disease, 21
brain disorders, 57
burns, 28, 41

cancer
  adjustment, 51–2
  child's understanding of, 83
  communication, 79–80
  coping strategies, 71

long-term, worries, 124
marital adjustment, 70
parents' knowledge of, 62
severity, 3
teasing at school, 112
see also leukaemia
cardiac catheterisation, 22
cerebral palsy
family resources, 67
maternal adjustment, 66
chronic disease
children's understanding of, 81–3
incidence, 2, 42, 48
severity, 4, 46, 50, 55, 56, 58, 63, 66, 75, 120
chronological age, 4, 58, 80
clinical practice, 6–8, 80
cleft palate, 2
see also birth defects
coeliac disease, 43
communication, 3, 9–10, 27, 70, 74–6, 78–92
competence, 47
compliance, 4, 9, 60, 93, 97
computer-based learning, 94
concepts
of the body, 85–6, 118–19
of death, 86, 87, 118–19
of hospital, 12
of illness, 4, 35, 81–4, 118–19
of pain, 34–6
of treatment, 12
congenital heart disease, *see* heart disease
coping, definition of 'good', 71
coping strategies, 10, 26, 36–8, 105–15
conclusions, 114–15
and degree of adjustment, 110
families, 70–2
future research needed, 111
general use of, 25
hospital admission, 23–5
interpersonal, 112–13
mastery-orientated/helpless, 113–14
parental adjustment and, 63–4
school-related, 113–14
theoretical approaches, 106–11; in adults, 108; in childhood, 109–11
see also stress
counselling, 39
cranial irradiation, 52

cystic fibrosis
adjustment, 57
child's understanding, 83
incidence and survival, 2, 42
marital relationship, 70
mother and, 62, 66
parents' knowledge of, 62

death
coping with, 71–2
dying child, 103–4
understanding of, 86, 87–8
developmental growth, effects of disease on, 5–6
developmental psychology
as an alternative approach, 116–18
concept of illness: changes in, 83–4; script approach, 90–1; stage approach, 845–8, 92
importance of, 3–4, 116
relationships, 59–60
research liaison with paediatrics, 126–7
stage approach: illness, 84–8, 92; pain, 34–5; problems of, 6, 118
structuralist/functionalist approach, 118–19
diabetes
adjustment, 53, 58
child's understanding, 81–2
coping strategies, 70
family interactions, 42, 43, 73, 76
family resources, 67, 68
incidence and survival, 2
intervention programmes, 93–4, 95, 97–8, 99
mother and, 62, 76
one-parent families, 77
parents' knowledge of, 62, 63
diabetic children, mother, 76
discipline, 76–7
divorce rate, 69–70
doctors
attitudes to, 12–13
pain associated with, 13
relevance of research to, 7–8, 126–7
dying child, 103–4
see also death

emotional contagion, 25

epilepsy
  control, 3
  mother's mental health, 62
  school achievement, 113

'faces' scale, 30
families
  adjustment, 4, 9, 61–77, 125–6
  communication and interaction, 74–5
  coping: definition of 'good', 71;
    general correlates, 71–2
  effects on, 1–2
  intervention programmes, 102
  one-parent, 77
  resources, 67–8
  see also father, mother, parents,
    siblings
father, 9
  diabetic children, 76
  importance of, 62, 66
  knowledge of disease, 62
  mental health, 62
  relationship with child, 66, 126
  see also families, parents
films, see video-films

gender, 124
grief and mourning, 71–2
group therapy, 102–3

haemophilia
  adjustment, 53–4, 58
  control, 3
  family resources, 43, 48, 67, 103
  incidence and survival, 2
  intervention programmes, 94, 103
  mother's mental health, 62
  pain, 28
handicapped children
  mother's mental health, 62
  siblings, 73
  social support network, 68
healthy children
  friendship with, 123
  hospital admission, preparation,
    18–20
  intervention programmes for, 101–2
heart disease
  incidence and survival, 2
  marital adjustment, 70

play therapy, 22
HIV infection, 54
hospital admission, 4, 8
  adolescents, 12–13
  conclusions, 27
  knowledge of hospitals, 12
  long-term disturbance, 16–17
  parents' role, 25–6
  preparation, 17–25, 27; acutely sick,
    21–5; well children, 18–20
  psychological impact, 14–17
  regression, 16
  stress of, 14
  tours prior to, 18, 25
  worries about, 11–12
  see also paediatric ward
hypnosis, 39–40
hypoglycaemia, 53

illness, concept of
  developmental changes in, 83–4
  general conclusions, 91–2
  script approach, 90–1
  stage approach, 84–8, 92
insulin, 42, 81
intelligence, 4–5, 121–2
intervention programmes, 10
  and adjustment, 93
  bereaved families, 102–4
  disease-related knowledge, 93–5
  general conclusions, 104
  parents, 102–3
  school-life, 100–2
  self-care skills, see self-care skills
  social skills, 98–100

juvenile diabetes, see diabetes
juvenile rheumatoid arthritis, see
    rheumatoid arthritis

KIDCOPE, 110
knowledge, 62, 101

leukaemia, 14
  child's understanding of death, 88
  coping strategies, 70–1
  incidence and survival, 2, 42, 52
  pain, 28
  parents' knowledge of, 62
  play therapy, 22

return to school-life, 100, 101
severity, 3
locus of control, 52
long-term effects, 124
lumbar puncture, 13

maladjustment, *see* adjustment, psycho-
    logical effects
marital relationship, 2, 59, 69–70
medical staff, attitudes to, 12–13
    see also doctors
meta-analysis, 27, 51
mother
    adjustment, 9, 63–4; of child, 59;
        resistance factors, 64, 65; risk factors,
        64–6
    knowledge of disease, 62
    as main carer, 61–2
    mental health, 62
    relationship with child, 125–6
    stress, 64, 66
    see also families, father, parents
muscular dystrophy, 2
myelination, 9

National Association for the Welfare of
    Children in Hospital (NAWCH),
    15
nurses, 13

obesity, 67
observation scale of behavioural distress,
    31
oncology, *see* cancer, leukaemia, bone-
    marrow aspirations, lumbar
    punctures
one-parent families, 77

paediatric ward
    changes in organisation, 16
    improvements in life on, 15–16
    and NAWCH, 15
    parents' role, 15–16
    Platt report (1959), 8, 15
    play-leaders and teachers, 16
    see also hospital admission
paediatricians, research and, 6–8, 126–7
    see also doctors
pain, 8–9, 13, 28–41

assessment, 29–34
coping strategies, 36–8
definition and understanding of, 34–6
developmental changes, 34
intervention strategies, 38–41; coping
    and stress-inoculation, 40–1;
    hypnosis, 39–40; puppet therapy,
    38–9; relaxation, 38
measurement, 29–33; behavioural,
    31–2; cognitive methods, 30–1;
    physiological, 33
and medical staff, 12–13
symptom-reporting, 36
undermedication, 29
parents
    adjustment, 63–4, 126; of child, 25–6;
        marital, 2, 69–70
    discipline, 76–7
    disease knowledge, 62–3
    and hospital admission, 25–6
    intervention programmes, 102–3
    on paediatric ward, 15–16
    single, 77
    support groups, 103
    see also families, father, mother,
        siblings
personality measurements, 123
phenylketonuria, 43, 68–9
physical disability, 49, 58, 62
Platt report (*Welfare of children in
    hospitals*), 8, 15
play therapy
    cardiac catheterisation, 22
    and hospital admission, 21–2, 27
    severe illness, disability, 22
play-leaders, and hospital admission,
    16, 21
problem-solving skills, 4, 102, 112
psychological effects, 9
    outcome measures, intelligence,
        121–2
    personality, 123
    research, approach of, 120–1
    social development, 122
    see also adjustment
punishment, 84, 88
puppet therapy, 24, 25, 38–9

regression, 16
relaxation therapy, 23–4, 38

renal disease, 56
  adjustment, 55
  incidence and survival, 2
research
  and clinical practice, 6–8
  general discussion, 3–6
resistance factors
  coping strategies, 70–2
  family resources, 67–8
  marital adjustment, 69–70
  siblings, 72–4
  social support network, 68–9
rheumatoid arthritis
  adjustment, 54–5
  family resources, 43, 67
  severity, 3
risk factors, 64–6

school, 100–2
  absenteeism, 113
  achievement, 113, 114
  hospital role-playing, 18–20
  phobia, 100
  stress, 113–14
school-based programmes, 18, 100–2
scripts, 89–91
self-care skills
  compensatory behaviour, 96–7
  external controlling, 97–8
  intervention, 96
  prevention, 96
siblings, 5
  adjustment, 72–4
  changed expectations of, 73
  differential parental treatment, 61,
    72–3
  of handicapped children, 73
  positive aspects of relationship, 74
  psychological reaction, 73–4
  see also families

sickle-cell anaemia
  adjustment, 56–7
  incidence and survival, 2
  school achievement, 113
social skills
  development, 122–3
  intervention programmes, 98–100
social support networks, 68–9, 71, 107
spina bifida, 2
  adjustment: child's, 57, 58; marital,
    70; maternal, 48, 62, 66
  family resources, 67
  incidence and survival, 2
  school achievement, 113
  social support networks, 68
stereotypes, 109
stress
  coping strategies, 37–8
  hospital-related, 4, 14
  parental, 64, 66
  school-related, 113–14
  social support network and, 68
  see also coping strategies
stress–inoculation model, 23–4, 40–1
symptom reporting, 36, 94

teachers, 16, 57, 73, 100–2
  see also schools
teasing, 113
temperament, 47, 109, 121
tonsillectomy, 16
transgression, 35

video-films, 20, 22–3, 24

Welfare of Children in Hospital,
  National Association, 15
Welfare of children in hospitals (Platt
  Committee), 8, 15